Darlan Rodrigues Macedo
Joselito N. Costa
Wendell M. S. Perinotto

Verminosis and eimeriosis in dairy goats in semi-arid Bahia

Darlan Rodrigues Macedo
Joselito N. Costa
Wendell M. S. Perinotto

Verminosis and eimeriosis in dairy goats in semi-arid Bahia

Parasite control strategies for small ruminants

ScienciaScripts

SUMMARY

ACKNOWLEDGMENTS

To my parents Deraldo and Lindaura, my sisters Ana Cléia and Luciana, who, even though they don't know exactly what I'm doing, support me in every moment and decision I make. Without you, nothing would be possible.

To my grandparents *(in memoriam)*, all my uncles and cousins, who encouraged me to continue on this path.

To Professor Joselito Nunes Costa, for his friendship, guidance, patience and trust in my ability. For the professional and personal example he sets for me and for showing me the way through books.

To Dr. Carmo Emanuel Almeida Biscarde, for his knowledge, advice and friendship. Thank you for always believing in me and showing me that I can be better every day.

To Professor Wendell Marcelo de Souza Perinotto, for his help in developing this work, learning and for opening the doors of the parasitology laboratory whenever I needed it.

To Professor Raul Rio Ribeiro, for the knowledge he imparted and for his trust and encouragement.

To the professors at the Federal University of Recôncavo da Bahia for their teaching, patience and for making this path possible.

To Danielle Nobre Santos Pinheiro, for her trust, friendship and for always being willing to help me.

To all the producers in the municipalities of Conceição do Coité, Valente and Sao Domingos, for their coexistence, friendship, trust in our work and for all the knowledge shared. You are living proof that "The sertanejo is, above all, a strong man". (Euclides da Cunha).

To Professor José Augusto Garcia, M.V. José Dantas Bitencuort, M.V. Bruno Cabirta, Agronomist Ricardo Miranda, all the teachers and colleagues from the technical course in agriculture at CETEP NE II in Ribeira do Pombal-BA, for their friendship and for believing in me.

To the friends I met during this journey, Caio Pereira, Saulo Cunha, Caio Freitas, Walber Varjao, Edivan Ferreira, Manuel Diran, Ricardo Santana (Riachao), Eduardo Guimaraes, Fernando Biscarde, Renata Machado, Marta Eloy, Sóstenes Apolo, Laura Nicole, Jéssica Santos, Fernanda Martins, Karolini Oliveira, Rosimere Santana, Ana Paula Abreu and Almir Rodrigues. Thank you for all your help and affection. You have undoubtedly made this journey less painful and more enjoyable.

To the University's civil servants and technicians, all my colleagues in the large animal clinic and other sectors of the UFRB. It has been a pleasure working with you.

To old and invaluable friends, for their help, encouragement and especially for allowing me to be part of their lives, Arnaldo Bastos, Francisco Sérgio, Gilson Rodrigues, Jariomar Cardoso (Max), José Màrcio, Ronaldo Macedo, Ricardo Santana, Célio Roberto, Fabrisio Campos, Hermênio Santana (Pita), Ana Paula Rodrigues, Edilza Almeida, Pedro Paulo Rodrigues, Armando Jesus and Luciana Bastos (*in memoriam*).

To my lovely daughter Livia, for her patience, understanding and love. To whom I apologize for these years of absence.

To all the people of Barrocao and Nova Esperança and so many other places, who helped me in some way and always cheered me on.

To God for guiding me with his divine strength, providing countless good things during this period, allowing me to see this journey through to the end and for always putting wonderful people in my life.

You don't know how far I walked to get here I walked miles and miles before I went to sleep I didn't doze off...

The most beautiful mountains I've climbed On dark, cold nights I've cried... Life teaches and time sets the tone...

Cidade Negra

SUMMARY

One of the factors that directly influences the success of parasite control is knowledge of the biology and epidemiology of parasites, and understanding these factors can help to establish more efficient strategies and methodologies. The aim of this study was therefore to diagnose gastrointestinal worms and eimeria, as well as to verify the profile and control practices used on goat farms in the Sisaleira region of Bahia and to describe the owners' perception of the importance of gastrointestinal parasites in goats. Data was obtained from 20 properties in the municipalities of Conceiçao do Coité, Sao Domingos and Valente. For the parasitological analysis, the animals were divided into two categories, under and over one year old. The feces were collected from the rectal ampulla of the animals and the OPG and OoPG techniques were used to quantify the estimated number of gastrointestinal helminths and *Eimeria sp.* in the herds, respectively. Semi-structured interviews were carried out to assess producers' perceptions, using a form drawn up by the authors. The OPG and OoPG showed that all the properties studied had parasitized animals. The results found in the analysis of the questionnaires made it possible to see that the properties were small, and that the predominant farming method was semi-intensive. This type of farming favors the maintenance of both worms and eimeria, since the animals spend some time together, due to the need for supplementation, thus facilitating the transmission of parasitic agents. Through this study, it can be concluded that the profile of the properties studied is in line with the regional reality, most of which are family subsistence farms with a small number of animals. In addition, most producers still have little knowledge of gastrointestinal parasites, especially eimeria, and as a result, the forms of control used for these diseases in the region are not sufficient. Therefore, other forms of control need to be implemented, especially in terms of management, given that even with the unfavorable climate for the cycles of these parasites, they still perpetuate themselves and cause serious problems in herds.

Keywords: Goats; worms; epidemiology.

1 - INTRODUCTION

The semi-arid northeastern region is known for its vegetation and especially for its climate, where rainfall is irregular and scarce, thus compromising the availability of fodder for much of the year. The animals of this region, especially the goat species, manage to withstand the harsh droughts by seeking their food in the caatinga (from the Tupi-Guarani: caa [forest]+tinga [white] made up of xerophilous and hyperxerophilous (sun-friendly) plants such as the cacti: mandacaru (*Cereus jamacaru*), xiquexique (*Pilosocereus gounellei*) and palm (*Opuntia and Nopalea*). Another plant of great importance in the region is sisal (*Agave sisalana*, figure 1), which as well as providing raw material for making various products (handicrafts), its by-products are a source of food for animals, making this plant the symbol of resistance and prosperity for the inhabitants of the Sisaleira region of Bahia.

Figure 1- Sisal (*Agave sisalana*).

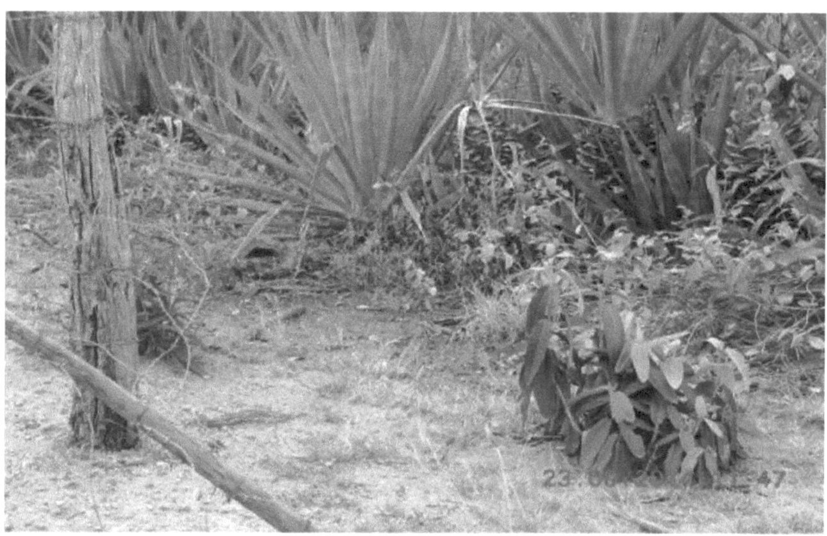

Source: Large Animal Clinic - UFRB.

The rearing of small ruminants in the semi-arid Northeast follows the history of its inhabitants, who for decades have used goat products such as meat, skin, milk and their derivatives as an important source of income, and for many, as a means of subsistence. Therefore, this activity stands out for playing an important socio-economic role in the region (COSTA JUNIOR et al., 2005; SIMPLICIO., 2006). Brazil has around 8.85 million goats, with the Northeast having approximately 8.1 million goats, with Bahia standing out in this scenario for having the largest goat herd in the country, with 2,360,683 head (IBGE, 2016).

These herds face serious health problems, especially eimeria in young animals and gastrointestinal worms in both young and adult animals (COSTA et al., 2009). These diseases are responsible for major losses in goat and sheep farming, resulting in the underdevelopment of young animals and low meat and milk production, as well as leading to the death of several animals, both young and adult.

Mild infections allow hosts to maintain an adequate immune response to the challenges posed by these nematodes, however, when these barriers are overcome, some strategies must be adopted so that, combined, they prevent the number of parasites from becoming pathogenic (HART., 2011; TORRES-ACOSTA et al., 2012).

The way to control worms on 100% of properties in the sisaleira region of Bahia is still the use of anthelmintics (PINHEIRO, 2015). However, the massive use of anthelmintic drugs increases the selection of strains resistant to these chemical compounds, which has been proven in the region, particularly with beef goats (BORGES et al., 2015).

Diagnosing these diseases in dairy goat herds in the Sisal region will allow us to understand the mechanisms by which these agents spread in these herds and to devise control strategies that suit the reality of the semi-arid region. Thus, the results of this study will help to determine the importance of gastrointestinal worms and eimeria in dairy goats in the Sisal-BA region, and to devise more efficient control strategies.

2 - LITERATURE REVIEW

2.1- - Main Gastrointestinal Parasites of Goats

Gastrointestinal endoparasitoses, such as worms and eimeria in goats, are a problem all over the world, especially in tropical regions, where the damage caused by these infections is more pronounced (VIEIRA, 2005).

The biggest obstacles to obtaining good zootechnical indices in goat breeding in extensive systems are gastrointestinal endoparasites (RINALDI & CRINGOLI, 2012). Among the nematodes that cause the greatest damage in small ruminant farming, either through delayed development or animal mortality, the following stand out: *Haemonchus spp., Trichostrongylus sp., Cooperia sp., Oesophagostomum spp. and Strongyloides papilosus* (BRITO et al., 2009*)*.

Another growing health problem in small ruminants is eimeriosis (SILVA et al., 2007), and its importance is due not only to the deaths, but also to the reduction in productivity, given that infected animals remain on the farm for longer to reach a desirable weight, thus increasing production costs (ANDRADE JÛNIOR et al., 2012; VIEIRA, 2005.

2.2- Main Etiological Agents of Verminosis and Eimeriosis

2.2.1- Etiology of gastrointestinal nematodes

The main parasites of importance to small ruminants belong to the order Strongylida, to which some superfamilies belong: Trichostrongyloidea, with the species*: Haemonchus contortus, Trichostrongylus axei,* parasites of the abomasum of ruminants and *Trichostrogylus columbriformis, Cooperia curticei, C. punctata*, parasites of the intestine of ruminants.

The genus *Oesophagostomum*, belonging to the Strongyloidea family, are nodular worms found in the large intestine of small ruminants. The Rhabditida order is also notable due to the prevalence in goat herds of the *Strongyloides papillosus* species, which are filariform worms found in the small intestine of ruminants (BOWMAN, 2010).

2.2.2- Etiology of Eimeriids

The genus *Eimeria* belongs to the subclass Coccidea and family Eimariidae. They have direct cycles and asexual and sexual forms of reproduction. The final product of sexual reproduction is the oocysts, which are peculiar to the genus and, after sporogony in the environment, present four sporocysts with two sporozoites each (FORTES, 1997).

Among the large number of *Eimeria* species that parasitize goats, some stand out for their prevalence and pathogenicity in goat herds in the Northeast region: *E. ninakohlyakimovae, E. arloingi, E. apsheronica* and *E. christenseni* (AHID et al., 2009).

Cattle, sheep and goats are parasitized by various species of *Eimeria*, however, these infections are species-specific (CHARTIER; PARAUD, 2012), but some species, such as *E. caprovina*, can also be found parasitizing the sheep species (AHID et al., 2009).

2.3- Evolutionary cycle of gastrointestinal nematodes and eimeriids

2.3.1- Evolutionary Cycle of Gastrointestinal Nematodes

The biological cycles are direct, with development starting from eggs that are thrown into the environment along with the feces, undergoing transformations that range from 16 to 32 cells, embryo and hatching in 1 or 2 days, resulting in a first-stage larva (L1), which feeds on bacteria present in the fecal bolus. This is followed by the first molt into a second-stage larva (L2), which is free-living and also feeds on microorganisms. This is followed by the second molt, which retains the sheath or cuticle from the previous stage and becomes an infective third-stage larva (L3). This cycle can be completed in 4-7 days from the embryonated egg, which is dependent on humidity and heat conditions. The L3 retains the cuticle from the previous larval stage, which in turn serves as protection against dissection. This results in a larva with infective power, which can migrate out of the fecal mass and then into the vegetation, especially when it finds suitable water, waiting for a susceptible host. The stage from egg to L3 is called the free-living stage. When the L3 is ingested by this host, it loses its cuticle in the abomasum and passes into the fourth stage (L4), initiating histotrophy in the abomasum by *Haemoncus sp and Trichostrongylus sp.* The next step is to pass into the adult stage (L5) or enter hypobiosis (BOWMAN, 2010) (Figure 2).

Figure 2- Biological cycle of the main gastrointestinal nematodes in goats.

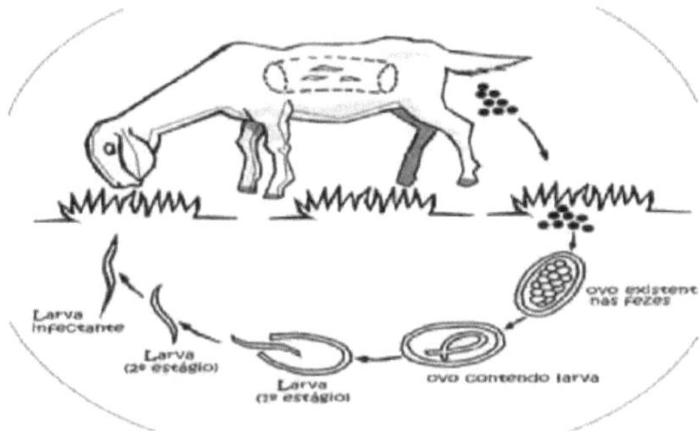

Source: (BOWMAN, 2010).

Trichostrongylus sp and *Oesophagostomum sp*, when they reach the adult stage, copulate and their females begin a daily oviposition of around 200 and 3,000 eggs per day, respectively (UENO and GONÇALVES, 1998), while *Haemonchus* has a much higher capacity than the others, with a daily oviposition capacity of 5,000 to 10,000 eggs (RADOSTITS et al, 2002; DIEHL et al, 2004). Images of *Haemonchus sp.* (Figure 3).

Figure 3- Adult specimens of *Haemonchus contortus* (A-B), (C) third-stage larvae and (D) specimens of *H. contortus* recovered from the necropsy of a goat.

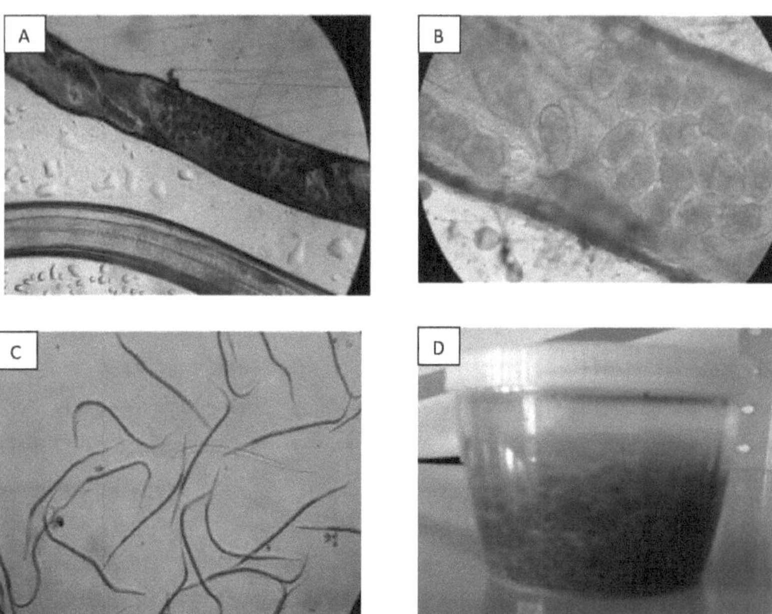

Source: UFRB Large Animal Clinic

The period between the ingestion of the infective larva and the detection of eggs in the feces of this host can be called the pre-patent period, which varies from species to species, being on average two to three weeks for most trichostrongylids (ALMEIDA et al., 2005; BOWMAN, 2010).

2.3.2- Evolutionary Cycle of Eimeriids

The life cycle of the genus *Eimeria* is considered to be direct, i.e. it only needs one host to complete its cycle, which includes three stages: sporogony, merogony and gametogony. After the non-sporulated and therefore non-infective oocysts are released into the feces, they undergo a sporulation phase in the environment, which gives them infective power. Sporulation takes place over 2-7 days and is dependent on temperature, oxygen and humidity. After sporulation, this sporulated oocyst now has four sporocysts inside, each with two sporozoites. Therefore, after ingesting a sporulated oocyst, it will release eight sporozoites through the operculum, which invade the lamina propria of the intestinal mucosa, where there is a change in shape and size, and it is now called a trophozoite, which releases numerous merozoites, which penetrate new healthy cells and produce the second generation of schizonts, which also produces another generation of merozoites. This phase, called merogony, is asexual and exponential and there can be several schizont generations, but two to five are the limit for most species of Eimeria. To complete the cycle, the merozoites invade new enterocytes and differentiate into male and female gametes (gametogonia) in the sexual phase, which give rise to oocysts (BOWMAN, 2010). (Figure 4).

Figure 4 - Biological cycle of *Eimeria* sp.

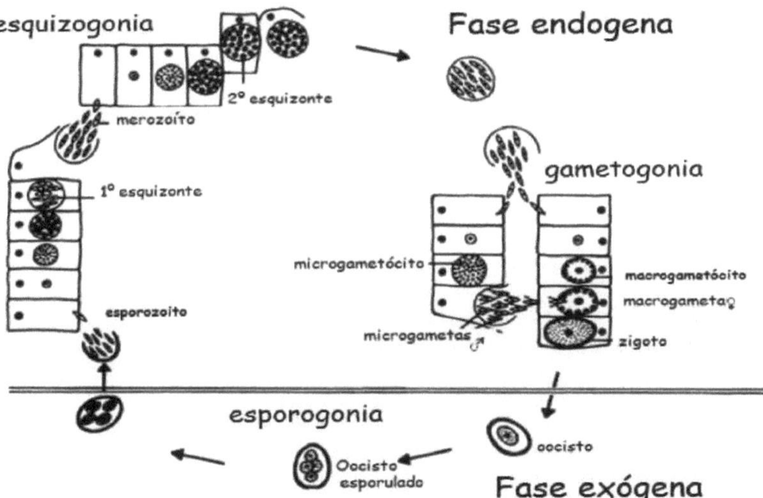

2.4- Epidemiology of Gastrointestinal Nematodes and Eimeriids

2.4.1- Epidemiology of gastrointestinal nematodes in goat farming

Infection by gastrointestinal nematodes is conditioned by climatic factors such as relative humidity (80 - 100%) and temperature (18 - 26°C), which play a decisive role in the survival of infective larvae in pastures (GASBARRE et al., 2001). In addition to these factors, conditions such as grazing areas where there is good soil cover by the pasture provide shade, which protects the larvae from desiccation and monthly rainfall rates above 50mm increase the chances of infection (BRAGHIERI et al., 2007).

What determines the infection of goats by gastrointestinal nematodes is the ingestion of the L3 together with the forage. In the semi-arid Northeast, as well as in other regions, the survival of these larvae ranges from 30 to 90 days (TORRES-ACOSTA & HOSTE, 2008). Goat feces in their sibalas format, when deposited during the dry season and at mild temperatures, remain intact, which guarantees the survival of larvae inside, which can reach 105 days (ALMEIDA et al., 2005).

Therefore, the survival of these larvae is dependent on the type of pasture, temperature, humidity, season and rainfall, the latter being considered the determining factor for larval development, especially in the northeast (RIET-CORREA et al., 2007). The survival rate varies from 42 to 56 days in spring, 70 to 84 days in summer, 112 to 126 in fall and 90 to 112 days in winter in southern Brazil (SOUZA et al., 2000). Another important factor is that these larvae have negative phototropism, so they tend to look for more favorable environments, i.e. they move away from the light and towards the ground, where they can penetrate, either by the action of rain or by voluntary movements (HOLASOVA et al., 1989). (Figure 5)

Figure 5- Goat droppings in the shape of sibalas (A), (B) Pasty droppings from goats fed a grain-rich diet, (C) Water reservoir and (D)

goat droppings near the vegetation on the banks of the reservoir.

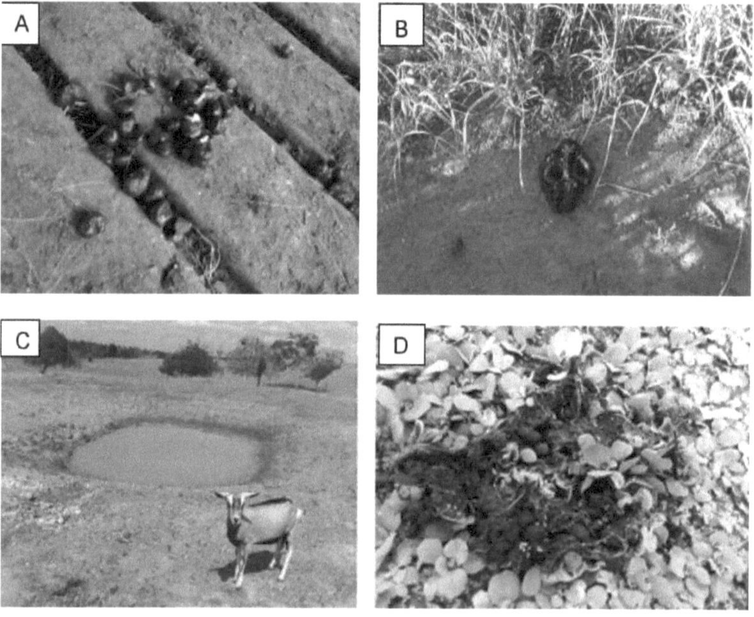

Larvae migrated out of the fecal pellet when rainfall exceeded 39 mm for goats and 28 mm for sheep. However, this migration was later for larvae from goat feces when compared to sheep feces, 49 and 21 days respectively. Most of the larvae are around 15 cm horizontally from the fecal mass. As far as vertical displacement is concerned, there is an influence of the size of the grass, with 80% of the larvae being found in the upper half of forage plants that are over 20 cm tall, being at least 12.5 cm high (ALMEIDA et al., 2005).

In tropical regions, endoparasitosis is a major issue in goat farming due to the damage it causes to production, as around 95% of goats are affected by some degree of parasitism (GITHIGIA et al., 2001). In the northeast of Brazil, studies show that more than 80% of the parasite load of small ruminants is made up of the *Haemonchus* genus (AROSEMENA et al., 1999).

Goats harbor a greater number of parasites during the rainiest periods of the year, probably due to the survival of the infective larvae (BRITO et al., 2009). Outbreaks of gastrointestinal worms in the semi-arid region are concentrated at the end of the rainy season and the beginning of the dry season and the disease affects young and adult animals, especially when pastures are overcrowded (COSTA et al., 2009).

The high levels of parasitic infection can partly be explained by the adoption of new production systems such as semi-intensive farming, which increases the possibility of infection and re-infection, the introduction of imported breeds which are more productive and less resistant to worms, the formation of pastures with grasses, which provide shade, thus avoiding the desiccation of eggs and larvae, and high stocking rates (COSTA et al., 2011).

Goats are more susceptible than sheep when both species graze together. This may be associated with the feeding habits that goats have developed over the years, preferring shrubs, thus making it difficult for them to come into contact with the infective larvae, which can hardly migrate to these shrubs and, as a result, these animals are less able to mount an adequate response to these helminths (COSTA JÚNIOR et al., 2005; TORRES-ACOSTA & HOSTE, 2008).

Most animals have chronic and subclinical infections, which makes it difficult to diagnose them, although infections are almost always mixed, i.e. gastric and intestinal nematodes parasitizing the same animal, although *Haemonchus contortus* is prevalent in more than 80% of worm cases (COSTA & VIEIRA, 1984; SILVA et al., 2011).

2.4.2- Epidemiology of Eimeriids

Eimeria occurs all over the world, mainly affecting young animals kept stabled without proper hygiene or those that graze in small areas, especially when they share these with adult animals. Due to the morphological similarities of the oocysts, it was believed that goats and sheep harbored the same species of *Eimeria*, however, it is accepted that the infection is species-specific, with the exception of *E. caprovina, E. pallida, E. punctata,* which have the power to infect both goats and sheep (ABO-SHEHADA & ABO-FARIEHA, 2003; AHID et al., 2009).

Coccidiosis is a disease responsible for significant intestinal changes, which can lead to a decrease in appetite and consequent underdevelopment, with a mortality rate of up to 10%, especially in dairy goats and lambs in confinement (MACIEL et al., 2006).

Infection is always oral-fecal due to contamination of food, water, teats, hair contaminated with feces or dust containing sporulated oocysts. They sporulate for 2-7 days and are dependent on temperature, oxygen and humidity. When sporulated, they can survive for up to two years in the environment, but temperatures above 35 °C, humidity below 25% and sunlight for four hours are fatal for some species. Infection can occur as early as the first week of life through the ingestion of sporulated oocysts acquired during feeding. The elimination of oocysts in the feces can appear from 15 days post-infection (RADOSTITS et al., 2002).

Poor hygiene in the facilities, which includes drinking and feeding troughs with feces, damp bedding, overcrowding of pastures by different categories, concomitant parasitism, stress and inadequate feeding programs, all lead to massive infections by intestinal coccidiosis. Young animals from 15 days to 11 months of age are the most susceptible and the ones that eliminate the most oocysts into the environment (COSTA et al., 2009), 2009). However, adult animals are important sources of environmental contamination by eliminating large quantities of oocysts, especially breeding animals in the mating season, lactating animals, pregnant animals and adult animals under high levels of stress, which can show clinical signs of the disease (BOMFIM & LOPES, 1994; VIEIRA et al., 1999).

2.5- Pathogenesis of the Main Gastrointestinal Nematodes and Steroids

2.5.1- Pathogenesis of gastric worms

The pathogenesis and severity of clinical signs are dependent on factors such as: (1) susceptible hosts, which include young animals, periparturient females, animals with nutritional compromise, immunity developed in previous contacts and high stress levels, (2) parasite load, species of nematodes involved, (3) environmental conditions favorable to the development and survival of larval stages in the pasture (VANDAMME & ELLIS, 2004; SADDIQI et al., 2011).

The *Haemonchus contortus* and *Trichostrongylus axei* species are important abomasal nematodes in small ruminants; however, *H. contortus* stands out from other parasites due to its high pathogenicity and prevalence in small ruminant herds (COSTA et al., 2009; GALLIDIS et al., 2012).

Due to the hematophagous habit in which a single specimen of *H. contortus* can draw about 0.05 mL of blood per day, massive infections by this species can trigger a hemodynamic imbalance in the host in which death can be the next step due to severe anemia, especially if poor nutrition or stress are involved (RADOSTITS et al., 2002; BOWMAN, 2010).

Both the L4 and the adults are hematophagous, so when the loss of these blood components exceeds the host's ability to produce them, the characteristic clinical signs of hemoncosis may appear. A striking feature would be the marked loss of blood components such as albumin, which leaks into the lumen of the abomasum and, subsequently, through the poor digestion and absorption of nutrients, characterizing hypoalbuminemia. Another important point would be "dyspepsia", when there is an increase in pepsinogen in the circulation, which occurs as a result of the inflammatory process of the abomasal mucosa due to the action of the parasites. This partially inhibits the production of hydrochloric acid (HCl), which is responsible for keeping the abomasal pH acidic, in the range of 2, which would be ideal for the conversion of pepsinogen into pepsin, the enzyme responsible for breaking down proteins. As a consequence, the destruction of bacteria and protozoa in the rumen is compromised, reducing their use as nutrients. Another element found in high concentrations is gastrin, which decreases reticulorum motility and consequently slows down the emptying of the abomasum, leading to partial anorexia, a common feature of parasitized animals. The sibalas are well formed and diarrhea only occurs when there is concomitant infection by intestinal nematodes (FOX, 1997; RADOSTITS et al., 2002; COSTA et al., 2009; SILVA, 2014).

Birgel et al (2014) showed that there may be a direct relationship between the intensity of the anemia and the globular volume, with the egg count per gram of feces (OPG) for the *Trichostrongyloidea* superfamily, mainly *Haemonchus sp.*, in which counts below 2000 eggs lead to mild anemia, while counts above 7000 eggs cause intense anemia. Animals fed diets low in protein are more vulnerable to the disease, showing more pronounced clinical signs than those fed diets high in protein (ACOSTA et al., 2006).

2.5.2- Pathogenesis of Intestinal Verminosis

The significant presence of nematodes, either in the lamina propria or in the intestinal lumen, causes alterations ranging from the loss of digestive/absorptive capacity due to the destruction of microvilli and replacement by scar tissue, to the loss of plasma proteins, permeability disorders and changes in peristalsis (HOSTE, 2001).

Trichostrongylus colubriformis infections are usually asymptomatic, but when they are present in large numbers they can cause serious problems for the host (ROCHA et al., 2008). The larvae that reach the small intestine migrate through the epithelium forming tunnels and, in severe cases, reach the lamina propria, leading to hyperemia, mucosal edema and villous atrophy, which contributes to a reduction in nutrient absorption. These larvae remain for a period of 10 to 12 days, from where they emerge into the intestinal lumen, causing capillaries to rupture in the process, which leads to the exudation of liquids leading to a hydro-electrolytic imbalance, culminating in hypoproteinemia and diarrhea (HOLMES, 1985; SILVA, 2014).

Oesophagostomum ssp, also known as ruminant nodular worms, is due to the parasitic larvae, which are histotrophic and induce a strong type IV inflammatory reaction, which can be responsible for acute cases of the disease, especially in previously sensitized hosts, leading to the encapsulation of these larvae, forming nodules in the intestinal wall. These nodules become caseous and calcified and can compromise the mechanical function of the intestine, however, when these larvae emerge they cause severe enteritis (RADOSTITS, et al., 2002; AMARANTE, 2005; BOWMAN, 2010).

Strongyloides papillosus infections are asymptomatic and in some cases mild, with neonates, immunocompromised animals and lactating females being the most susceptible. However, infections with this parasite can cause serious illness in goats, even in relatively mild infections. Experimentally, infections with larval doses of *S. papilosus* have been shown to cause the death of some goats. The main route of transmission is transmammary in which the larvae from an initial infection migrate to deeper tissues, passing into the milk and colostrum and on to their offspring (BOWMAN, 2010).

2.5.3- Pathogenesis of Eimeriosis

The intestinal epithelium is made up of absorptive, goblet and endocrine cells, originating from undifferentiated cells that rest on the basal membrane covering the lamina propria (DUKES, 2014). When these cells are destroyed in the infection process, they are replaced by smooth cells with a low absorption capacity (LIMA, 2004).

After a host has ingested sporulated *Eimeria* oocysts, the latter, through enzymatic processes, release the sporozoites, which in turn cause destruction of the intestinal microvilli in their multiplication process (FOREYT, 1990), giving rise to schizonts, structures containing hundreds of merozoites, which emerge through the ruptured cells to infect new cells, thus accelerating the process of epithelial degeneration. This process leads to loss of microvilli and destruction of the lamina propria (DAUGSCHIES & NAJDROWSKI, 2005).

2.6- Clinical Findings of Gastrointestinal Verminosis and Eimeriosis

2.6.1- Clinical Findings of Gastric Verminosis

The clinical findings of gastric worms can be classified into three forms: In the acute form, there are signs of dehydration, lethargy, dull and shiny hair, weight loss and, above all, anaemia, which can be seen when the conjunctival, gingival and vaginal mucous membranes are extremely pale) compensatory tachycardia, normal stools and partial anorexia in most cases. The chronic form, in most cases, is characterized by its subclinical aspect, however, some animals present submandibular edema and possible ventral edema, due to the loss of proteins, especially albumin (RADOSTITS et al., 2002; CHAGAS, 2009; MOLENTO, 2009; VIEIRA, 2009). Images of goats with clinical signs of gastric worm disease (Figure 6).

Figure 6- Goats with characteristic signs of anemia, in (A) pale oral mucosa, (B) hypochromic conjunctival mucosa, (C) submandibular edema, (D) blood taken from a goat with normal VG for the species and (E) blood taken from the goat in image C.

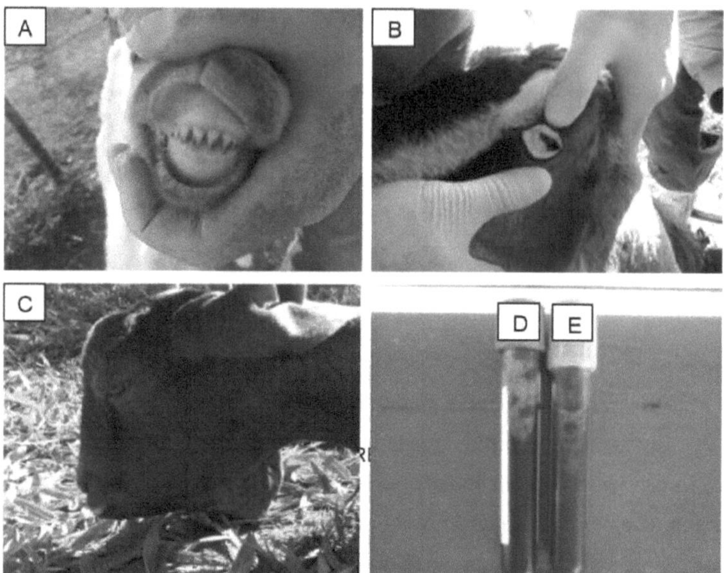

Anemia varies in its degree of intensity, which is directly related to the infectious load, as evidenced by the results of the egg count per gram of feces (OPG). Thus, it can be mild, moderate or intense, with globular volume values varying from 22-25%, 14-21% and 7-12% respectively, and the results found for OPG varying from 1183± 1975, 1750 ± 2818 and 8407 ±1305. The "PROC GLM" command was used to calculate the variance, and the contrast between the means was analyzed using the Student's t-test, with significance levels equal to 5% ($p \leq 0.05$) (BIRGEL et al., 2014). (BIRGEL et al., 2014).

2.6.2- Clinical findings of intestinal worms

Severe infections with *Trichostrongylus ssp., Oesophagostomum ssp., Cooperia ssp. and Trichuris ssp.* cause watery diarrhea with a dark green color, leading to weakness and sometimes prostration, especially in animals on a deficit diet or under stress. Due to the diarrhea, there is an accumulation of feces adhered to the tail or wool, which dries out and forms rattling structures when the animal is moving. Images of goats with characteristic signs of intestinal worms (Figure 7).

Figure 7- Goats showing characteristic clinical signs of intestinal worms. In (A)

Feces adhered to the tail of a goat, (B) Profuse diarrhea in a goat.

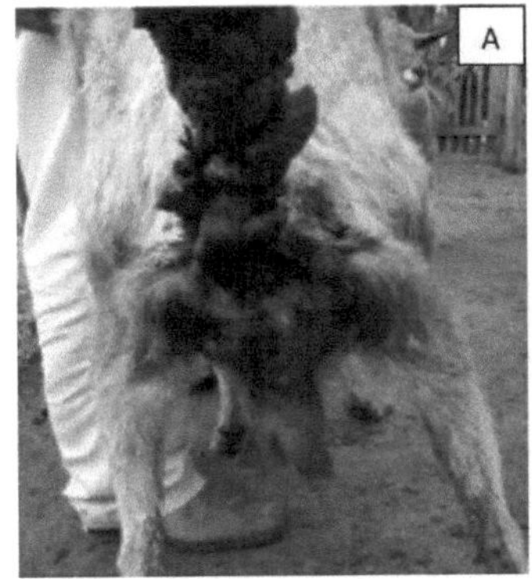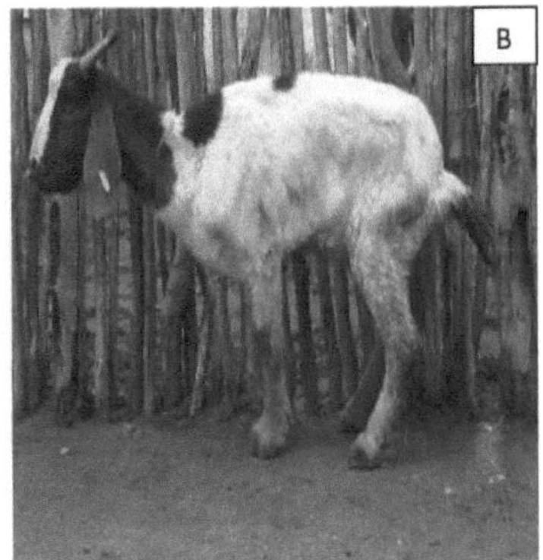

Source: Large Animal Clinic - UFRB

The result found in the OPG may be lower than expected, due to the fact that the feces are liquefied and the eggs are diluted in relation to the fecal volume (BOWMAN, 2010).

The clinical signs observed in animals experimentally infected with *Strongyloides papillosus* larvae were inappetence, cachexia, weakness, emaciation, dehydration, anemia, respiratory alterations and nervous symptoms. Necropsy findings included histopathological lesions in the spinal cord and brain, suggesting that *S. papilosus* may be more pathogenic than previously reported (PIENAAR, 1999).

2.6.3- Clinical Findings of Eimeriosis

Goats suspected of having eimeriosis may show a false negative result when counting oocysts per gram of feces (OoPG), or an insignificant result, especially if the fecal material is collected at the same time as the asexual reproduction phase (schizogony), when no oocysts are produced, or even after the peak elimination of these oocysts (gametogony) during sexual reproduction has passed (RADOSTITS, et al., 2002).

The clinical signs presented are characterized by apathy and anorexia, due to the thinning of the intestinal mucosa, which compromises the absorption of nutrients, as well as a certain loss of blood and organic fluids, which can lead to hypoproteinemia and anemia. The feces eliminated range from pasty to diarrheal, and from yellow-green to dark and fetid with or without the presence of blood, prostration, tenesmus with consequent rectal prolapse, dehydration and death of some animals, thus characterizing an acute condition. However, the most common form is subacute, in which there is mild diarrhea, slight apathy and low weight gain, making it subclinical. (Figure 8)

Figure 8- (A) Kids with characteristic signs of diarrhea, in (B) kids diagnosed with *eimeria*, in image (C) kid with signs of apathy cachexia and in (D) kid diagnosed with high counts of *Eimeria* oocysts, but without signs of diarrhea.

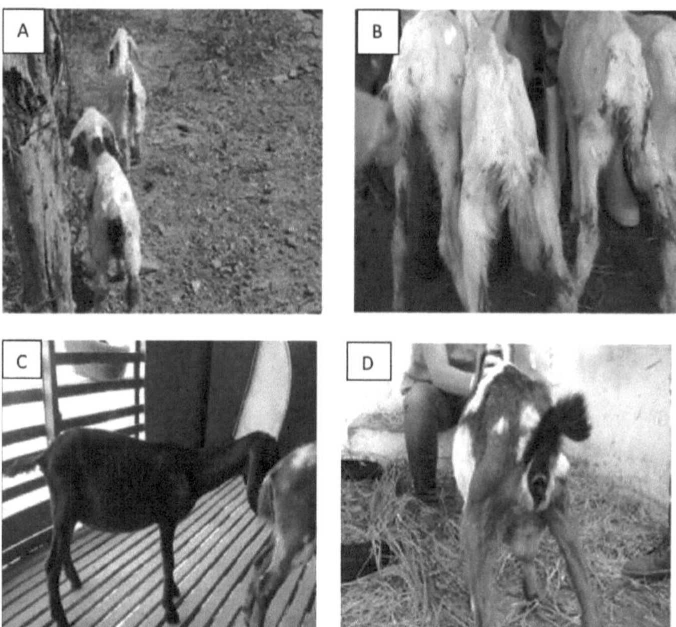

Source: Large Animal Clinic - UFRB

2.7- Diagnosis of gastrointestinal nematodes and Eimeriids

According to Smith (2006), infections resulting from the action of nematodes in small ruminants can be considered a clinical syndrome, since diarrhea, anemia, weight loss and shaggy hair are not specific to worms, since infectious agents, poor nutrition, mineral deficiency and plant poisoning can present the same symptoms (VIEIRA, 2008).

2.7.1- Egg count per gram of feces (OPG)

Carried out according to the technique of Gordon and Whitlock (1939) modified by Ueno & Gonçalves (1998), its advantages are the speed of diagnosis and the low cost of carrying out the examination, which can be done individually or by sampling the herd. This technique makes it possible to identify eggs mainly from the Strongylida order.

2.7.2- Oocyst count per gram of feces (OoPG)

Performed according to the technique of Gordon and Whitlock (1939) modified by Ueno & Gonçalves (1998), it is also easy to perform, however, care must be taken when interpreting it, since the technique can produce false negative results, inherent to the phase that the parasites are in (schizogony) where there is no production of oocysts (RADOSTITS et al.,

2002).

2.8- - Treatment of gastrointestinal worms

Treatment with anthelmintics is still the most common method used by farmers, and various active ingredients are used. The main groups are: benzimidazoles (Albendazole, Fenbendazole), macrocyclic lactones (Ivermectin), Imidazothiazoles (Levamisole Hydrochloride), salicylanilides (Closantel) (BORGES, 2003). In 2009, the first amine-acetonitrile derivative (Monepantel) was launched, followed by the second derivative of this molecule, in combination with a macrocyclic lactone (Abamectin) and derquantel (GEORGE et al., 2012). Different doses of anthelmintics for goats and sheep (table 1) Main anthelmintics available on the market (annexes 1, 2, 3, 4, 5 and 6)

Table 1 - Commercial broad-spectrum anthelmintics at different doses for goats and sheep.

	Dose mg/kg	Dose mg/kg	
Active ingredient	Sheep	Goats	Via adm.
Thiabendazole	50	100	Oral
Albendazole	5	10	Oral, Intra-ruminal
Mebendazole	15	30	Oral
Fenbendazole	5	10	Oral, Intra-ruminal
Oxfendazole	5	10	Oral, Intra-ruminal
Febantel	5	10	Oral, Intra-ruminal
Netobimin	7,5	15	Oral
Levamisole	7,5	12	Oral, Subcutaneous
Morantel	6	10	Oral
Ivermectin	0,2	0,3	Oral, Subcutaneous and Topical
Doramectin	0,2	0,2	Subcutaneous
Moxidectin	0,2	0,2	Oral, subcutaneous
Eprinomectin	0,5	1,0	Typical

Source: Torres-Acosta & Hoste (2008)

2.8.1- - Strategic treatment

This form of treatment recommends four dewormings a year, the first at the start of the dry season, the second sixty days later, the third in the penultimate month of the dry season and the fourth in the middle of the rainy season. This method is based on the knowledge that larvae survive less in the environment during the dry season, whereas during the rainy season they migrate more to the forage and subsequently become infected (COSTA & VIEIRA, 1994). However, this practice can accelerate the appearance of AR, which puts the control of worms at risk, since the entire herd is dewormed (CHARLES et al., 1989; KAPLAN et al., 2004; MOLENTO, 2004).

2.8.2-   -Selective treatment

Resistant animals contaminate pastures less than susceptible animals, which have egg counts per gram of feces (OPG) 4.1 times higher than resistant animals, with native breeds being more resistant (BASSETO, 2009).

The principle of selective treatment consists of understanding that 20 to 30% of a herd is home to 70 to 80% of the herd's adult parasite population. Therefore, identifying these animals and administering an antihemitic medication only to them, thus increasing the population in "Refuge", i.e. the portion of nematodes that have not come into contact with chemical products, thus reducing the risks of AR (RINALDI & CRINGOLI, 2012; HART, 2011).

The most widely used selective treatment is the FAMACHA method, a word derived from the initials of its creator Faffa Malan, plus the initials of the English word (chart) which means card. On this chart, there are five shades of 1, 2, 3, 4 and 5, and the colors range from bright red (1) to almost white (5), so there is an inverse relationship with the hematocrit values, which range from 35, 25, 20, 15 and 10%, respectively for groups 1 to 5 (VAN WYK, 2002).

In the Northeast of Brazil, *Haemonchus spp. is* the most frequent nematode and is responsible for major losses in production, with outbreaks of parasitosis being very common as a result of its action. Therefore, any parasite control program in northeastern Brazil should aim to control *Haemonhus spp* (COSTA et al., 2009). Because the FAMACHA method was developed with sheep, when it is used with goats it is necessary to wait around 8 seconds, since capillary filling is slower, whereas in sheep it is done immediately, requiring a different interpretation (REIS, 2004).

The disadvantage of this method is that it is only suitable for worms caused by hematophagous nematodes (VILELA et al., 2008).

The FAMACHA method, when combined with other techniques, makes it possible to know and select animals that are resistant to parasitosis, as well as resilient animals, which should be eliminated from the herd, since they do not show obvious signs of parasitosis, but contribute to the dissemination of large quantities of helminth eggs. However, if used correctly, it is possible to identify and treat only animals that really need treatment, increasing the population in "Refugia" and reducing production costs (MOLENTO et al., 2004).

Vilela et al (2008), working with FAMACHA in goats in the semi-arid region of Paraíba, concluded that goats only need to be treated when they have mucous membranes compatible with grade four.

Table 2 - Information contained in the FAMACHA card, degree of anemia and conjunctival coloration, corresponding to the globular volume (VG) and attitude to be taken with regard to the treatment of the animals.

Grade	Coloring	Variation doVG (%)	Attitude Clinic	
1	Robust red	> 28	Do Not Treat	Figure 9 - FAMACHA
2	Pinkish red	23 a 27	Untreated	
3	Pink	18 a 22	Treatment	
4	Pale pink	13 a 17	Treatment	
5	White	< 12	Treatment	

Source: Van Wyk; Bath (2002).

2.8.3- -Tactic treatment

This treatment recommends the use of dewormers when conditions favor environmental contamination, such as after heavy rains and also taking into account the physiological state of the animals such as: in animals just after weaning, before the mating season and in peripartum (COSTA et al., 2011).

2.8.4- -Eimeriosis treatment

Chemical compounds act in different ways, depending on their chemical nature.

Sulphamides are widely used to control and treat coccidiosis, however, their mechanism of action is limited to schizogony, which is the asexual phase of *Eimeria sp.* (VIEIRA, 2005; SIDDIKI et al., 2008; YOUNG et al., 2011).

Toltrazuril acts on all intracellular stages, i.e. both schizogony (asexual phase) and gametogony (sexual phase) (ALTREUTHER et al., 2011).

It should be noted that the infection is self-limiting, i.e. recovery is expected over a few days, especially if hygiene or management conditions improve (VIEIRA, 1996).

2.9- -Resistance to anthelmintics (RA)

The phenomenon of AR is the remarkable ability of a given population of parasites to survive doses of anthelmintics that could be lethal to susceptible populations. This AR can be lateral when it occurs with products from the same group, cross when it involves two drugs from different groups and multiple when it involves more than two pharmacological bases (VIEIRA, 2008; TORRES- ACOSTA & HOSTE, 2008; MOLENTO, 2005).

AR is widespread in goat herds in various states and regions of Brazil (MOLENTO, 2004), with some factors standing out: the indiscriminate use of antiparasitic products; the use of underdoses, which can occur due to the inaccuracy of the animals' body weight; the administration of doses recommended for sheep and not for goats, since goats metabolize anthelmintics more quickly than sheep; the very rapid alternation of pharmacological bases and the introduction of animals that harbour resistant populations. (TORRES-ACOSTA & HOSTE, 2008; COSTA et al., 2011).

The efficacy of antihemintics can be assessed by the test to reduce egg counts in feces (TRCOF), comparing the results before and after treatment with an antiparasitic (DEMELER et al., 2010). This test should be carried out once a year to monitor the effectiveness of the products and replaced when it is below 80% (FORTES & MOLENTO, 2013). The collection period after treatment is a decisive factor in the success of the technique since each product acts in a particular way on the animal organism. It is suggested that the collection of feces after treatment should be: 3-7 days for levamisole, 8-10 days for Benzimidazoles, 14-17 days for Macrocyclic Lactones, 21 days for Moxidectin and when more than one base is being used, samples should be taken after 14 days (COLES et al., 2006).

In goat herds raised in the extensive system in Rio Grande do Norte, post-treatment TRCOF found efficacy of 43% to 100% and 29% to 100% for ivermectin and albendazole, respectively (COELHO et al., 2010).

Similar results were obtained in surveys of anthelmintic resistance in the state of Ceará, on commercial goat farms, when 87%, 75% and 37% resistance to oxfendazole, levamisole and ivermectin were found, respectively (MELO et al., 2003).

In the state of Pernambuco, anthelmintic resistance was found in goat herds treated with albendazole, ivermectin and levamisole, with the percentages of efficacy varying between 11 and 61%, 14 and 76% and 67 and 89% respectively, while moxidectin was recommended for its efficacy of over 95% (LIMA et al., 2010).

Studies carried out in the municipality of Cansançâo in the sisaleira region of Bahia found anthelmintic resistance to albendazole, levamisole, ivermectin, moxidectin and closantel in goat herds in in vivo and in vitro tests (BORGES et al., 2013).

Sprengner et al (2013) evaluated the efficacy of levamisole phosphate in goats and sheep in the state of Paranà, with different doses: 4.75, 6.75 and 9 mg/kg of weight orally, and concluded that the product was not effective in goats in any of the treatments, however, for sheep, the doses of 6.75 and 9 mg/kg were efficient.

In a field study carried out in Brazil with sheep, resistance to monepantel was found, which was also suggested in studies in Australia and Uruguay. The results of the TRCOF and the critical test were 18.51% and 24.62% respectively, which is well below the minimum 80% recommended by MAPA. It is important to note that the management adopted on the property was deworming every two months (BERGAMASCO et al., 2015).

Cesar et al (2011) observed that it was possible to recover the efficacy of some anthelmintics in sheep, depending on an appropriate combination of drugs with different mechanisms of action and not needing to increase the dose. The efficacy of the eleven (11) bases used alone ranged from -35 to 68%, and when combined the result ranged from 64 to 99% (Tables 3 and 4).

Table 3- Treatments evaluated in the target flock of sheep in this **study.**

Groups (n=15) and treatments	Dose (mg/kg)[ii]	Classes a	Trade name, manufacturer
G1. Moxidectin 1% (Double the dose)	0,4	Milbemycin[b]	Cydectin sheep, Fort Dodge
G2. levamisole Phosphate 22.3% (Double the dose)	9,0	Imidazothiazole	Levamisol F, Vetbrands
G3. Moxidectin 1%	0,2	Milbemycin[b]	Cydectin sheep, Fort Dodge
levamisole phosphate 22.3%	4,5	Imidazothiazole	Levamisol F, Vetbrands
G4. Moxidectin 1%	0,2	Milbemycin[b]	Cydectin sheep, Fort Dodge
Disophenol 20%	10,0	Nitrophenol	Dysphenol 20%, IBASA
G5. Moxidectin 1%	0,2	Milbemycin[b]	Cydectin sheep, Fort Dodge
Trichlorfon 10%	100,0	Organophosphate	BevermexJRFA
G6. Moxidectin 1%	0,2	Milbemycin[b]	Cydectin sheep, Fort Dodge
Closantel 10%	10,0	Salicylanilide	Diantel, IRFA
G 7 levamisole phosphate 22.3%	4,5	Imidazothiazole	Levamisol F, Vetbrands
Trichlorfon 10%	100,0	Organophosphate	Bevermex, IRFA
G8. Moxidectin 10%	1,0	Milbemycin[b]	Onyx, Fort Dodge

[a] All parenterally, subcutaneously, except o Closantel 10% (via orai).

[b] Macrocyclic lactone.

Source: Alfredo Skrebsky Cesar et al., 2011.

Table 4- Percentage of each of the five genera of gastrointestinal nematodes - *Haemonchus* spp. (*Haem.*), *Trichostrongylus* spp. (*Trich.*), *Ostertagia* spp. (*Ostert.*), *Cooperia* spp. (*Coop.*), *Oesophagostomum* spp. (*Oesoph.*) - **recovered before** (D0) and 12 days after *(D12) the antiparasitic treatments.*) - recovered from cultures of larvae in sheep feces collected before (D0) and 12 days after (D12) antiparasitic treatments, and percentage reduction (PR), for each genus, calculated by RESO FECRT 4.0.

Groups (n=15) and treatments	*Haem. (%)*		*Trich. (%)*		*Osteit (%)*		*Coop. (%)*		*Oesoph. (%)*	
	DO	D12(PR)	DO	D12(PR)	DO	D12(PR)	DO	D12(PR)	DO	D12(PR)
G1. Moxidectin 1% (double the dose)	78	52(93)r[a]	4	40(0) R[a]	O	2(0)R	18	6(96)S[a]	O	O(NC)[b]
G2. Phosph. lev.[c] 22.3%	46	14(95)r	16	80(14)R	16	4(96)3	20	2(98)3	2	0(100)3

(double the dose)

G3. Moxidectin 1% + phosph. lev. 22.3%	68	6(99)S	4	91 (O)R	20	3(99)3	8	O(lOO)S	O	O (NC)
G4. Moxidectin 1% + d isophenol 20%	54	6(1 OOJS	10	86(89)R	20	4(1 OOJS	16	4(100)S	O	O (NC)
G5. Moxidectin 1% + trichlorfon 10%	80	26(97)S	2	48(0)R	2	20(6)R	16	6(96)8	O	O (NC)
G6. Moxidectin 1% + Closantel 10%	60	4(99)S	24	86(38)R	O	6(0)R	12	O(WO)S	6	2(94)r
G7. Light phosphate 22.3% + trichlorfon 10%	62	8(95)S	8	62(0)R	4	18(0)R	26	8(89)R	O	4(0)R
G 8. Moxidectin 10%	58	47(83)R	O	47(0)R	2	6(35)R	40	O(WO)S	O	O (NC)

[a] r = low resistance, R = resistant, S = Susceptible.

[b] NC = not calculated.

[c] Lev. phosphate = levamisol phosphate.

Source: Alfredo Skrebsky Cesar et al., 2011

Another technique used is stool culture (coproculture), according to Roberts & O'sullivam (1950), which makes it possible to identify the third-stage larvae of strongylids, classifying them by percentage into their respective genera (UENO & GONÇALVES, 1998).

3 - CONTROL

3.1- Control of gastrointestinal worms

There are various parasite control techniques, ranging from herd and pasture management, rotational grazing, biological control, nutrition, genetic selection, verification of the efficiency of anthelmintics and knowledge of parasite epidemiology. However, it is of fundamental importance for breeders and technicians to understand that methods which rely exclusively on the use of anthelmintics have proved to be unsustainable, and that integrated parasite control is therefore an excellent alternative, especially selective treatment and the selection of more resistant animals (MOLENTO, 2005; CEZAR et al., 2008; TIRABASSI et al., 2013).

Simple examples of control measures are: hygiene of the facilities, including feeders and drinkers, avoiding constant contact between animals and feces, building manure pits or giving feces a correct destination, avoiding overcrowding, deworming animals acquired from other properties, separating animals by category, weighing animals and using correct doses, fasting for 12 hours for oral products and providing only water up to six hours after deworming (VIEIRA, 2008).

Copper oxide in capsules has shown promise, however, only for the control of gastric worms (GONÇALVES & ECHEVARRIA, 2004). Since *Haemonchus spp.* is the main cause of parasitic outbreaks in the Northeast, any control program should be based on the control of this parasite (COSTA et al., 2009).

Therefore, the FAMACHA and OPG method should be adopted, with the aim of selective treatment, since it makes it possible to identify so-called resistant animals in the herd, which have the ability to mount a more efficient immune response, in which the host limits or prevents the development of the parasite, leading to a decrease in egg production, slowing down the growth of parasites or eliminating existing parasites (TORRES-ACOSTA & HOSTE 2008; BOWMAN, 2010; CHAGAS et al., 2013). Resilient or tolerant animals are those that are able to live with the parasites and do not show clinical signs of infection, however, they do not prevent the production of parasite eggs, thus contributing to the contamination of pastures (TORRES-ACOSTA & HOSTE 2008).

Resistant animals contaminate pastures less than susceptible animals, which have egg counts per gram of feces (OPG) 4.1 times higher than resistant animals, with native breeds being more resistant (BASSETO, 2009). Another important measure is to use TRCOF and co-culture to evaluate the effectiveness of the products and, through larval culture, to identify the genera present on the property (CHAGAS et al., 2013).

3.2- Eimeriosis control

Several studies carried out in goat herds in the Northeast have confirmed the diagnosis of Eimeria. However, it is difficult to control this disease because most animals carrying parasites of the genus *Eimera spp.* do not show specific clinical signs of the disease (AHID et al., 2009).

It is important to understand that eimeriosis is not just an individual problem, but a herd problem, due to the high possibility of animals coming into contact with the oocysts. In this context, it is necessary to rigorously sanitize the facilities, feed the animals properly, keep stress levels low, separate affected animals for treatment and use anticoccidial drugs preventively (LIMA, 2004; PUGH, 2004).

The form of control most farmers still use is antibiotics and other coccidiostats mixed into the feed, especially ionophores, decoquinate, sulphas and amprolium, which also act only on schizogony (VIEIRA, 2005; SIDDIKI et al, 2008; YOUNG et al., 2011).(Annex 7) However, decoquinate has the power to inhibit the sporulation of oocysts (DEL CACHO et al., 2006).

4 - OBJECTIVES

4.1- - General Objective

Determine the occurrence of gastrointestinal worms and eimeria in goat herds in the region and implement control measures.

4.2- - Specific Objectives

-To evaluate the profile of the farms and the producers' perception of the importance and control techniques for verminosis and eimeriosis.

-Characterize the relationship between farming systems and farm size with OPG and OoPG results.

-Identify possible flaws in health management.

-Evaluate the methods used to control worms and eimeria.

5 - MATERIAL AND METHODS

5.1- EXPERIMENTAL DESIGN

5.1.1 - Sample collection site

The crops were harvested in the cities of Conceiçao de Coité, Sao Domingos and Valente in the sisaleira region of Bahia, where the predominant biome is the caatinga. During the period of the experiment, the average temperature ranged from 19°C to 34°C and the average annual rainfall was 550 mm (IBGE, 2016). The data was obtained from 20 rural properties distributed in the three municipalities that make up an important dairy basin in the region, where so far there are two dairies (Ouro Verde and Apaeb), which together process approximately 3000 liters of milk/day.

5.1.2 - Animals

We used goats of the Saanen, Pardo alpina and mixed breeds (Figure 10), raised in extensive, intensive and semi-intensive systems. The animals were clinically assessed by a veterinarian from the work team, following the specific recommendations for the species, as well as age estimation through dental arch analysis following the recommendations of Pugh (2004).

The animals were divided into groups according to age, as follows:

Group 1: Animals under 1 year old;

Group 2: Animals over 1 year old.

Figure 10- Goats on a property in the municipality of Valente.

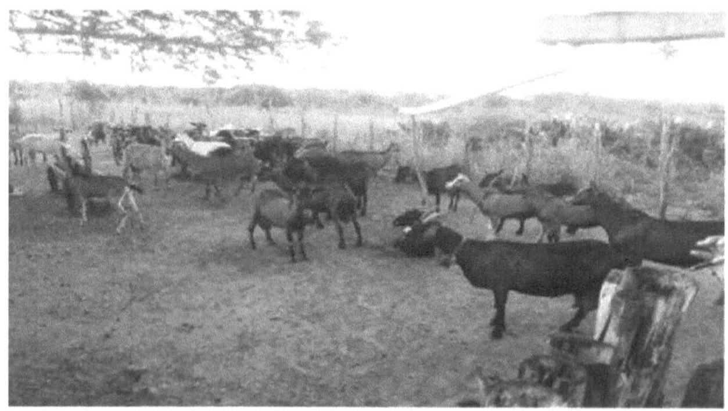

Source:Large animal clinic-UFRB

5.1.3 - Stool collection and coproparasitological tests

For the parasitological analysis, the animals on the farms were divided into two categories, under and over one year old. The feces were collected directly from the rectal ampulla of the animals, and each property collected them in a *pool* for each category mentioned above. Once the samples had been obtained and identified, they were taken to the Parasitology and Parasitic Diseases laboratory at the Federal University of Recôncavo da Bahia in isothermal boxes containing ice. To quantify the parasite load of gastrointestinal helminths and *Eimeria sp.* in the flocks, the OPG and OoPG techniques were used, respectively, according to Gordon and Whitlock (1939) with modifications by Ueno and Gonçalves (1998). (Figure 11) In order to check for possible predisposing factors to helminthiasis and eimeria, the OPG and OoPG results were divided into two categories, < 800 and ≥ 800 for gastrointestinal helminth eggs and < 2000 and ≥ 2000 for *Eimeria* sp. oocysts, respectively, according to Jùnior et al. (2005).

Figure 11- Material used to carry out the OPG and OoPG coproparasitological tests.

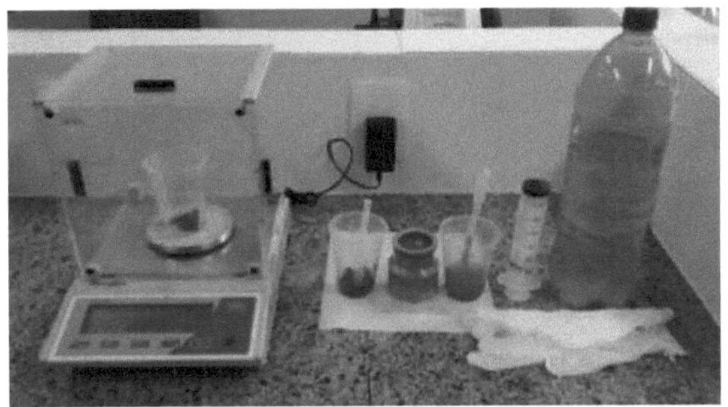

Source: Large Animal Clinic - UFRB.

In order to gain a better understanding of the profile of these farms, a questionnaire (appendix 8) was administered to the producers, with the aim of assessing their perception of the importance of and techniques for controlling worms and eimeria, identifying possible flaws in health management, and evaluating the methods used to control worms and eimeria.

5.1.4 Statistical analysis

The data obtained by counting eggs and oocysts per gram of feces among the different categories was calculated by analysis of variance (ANOVA), followed by the Tukey test at 5% significance, using the Instat 3.0 program. The answers were categorized using "content analysis" (MINAYO, 1993), in order to draw up a profile of the producers' perception of gastrointestinal helminths in goats. In addition, analysis of possible risk factors for helminthiasis and eimeriosis was carried out using Fisher's Exact Test, also using the Instat 3.0 program, and multivariate analysis to associate clinical signs with parasite load, using the R program.

6 - RESULTS

The quantitative analysis of gastrointestinal helminth eggs (OPG) and *Eimeria* sp. oocysts (OoPG) showed that all the properties studied had parasitized animals. When checking the parasite profile between young goats under 12 months old and adults over a year old, a higher count of helminth eggs from the trichostrongyloidea superfamily was observed in the adult animals, but with no significant difference (Table 5). In addition, it was possible to see a significant increase (*p* 0.0001) in relation to the established ranges of OPG < 800 and ≥ 800 (table 5), in the two categories evaluated, indicating high parasitism in the region's animals.

The results of the OPG, OoPG and questionnaire data are shown in tables 5, 6, 7, 8, 9, 10, 11 and 12.

Table 5. Egg count per gram of feces (OPG) of helminths of the Trichostrongyloidea superfamily, in leiteira goat farms in the semi-arid region of Bahia.

	OPG < 800	OPG ≥ 800	p-value
Animals up to 12 months	257 ± 222 aA (n = 10)	1,514 ± 452 aB (n = 7)	0,0001
Animals ≥ 12 months	258 ± 226 aA (n = 10)	2,809 ± 2004 aB (n = 10)	0,0001
p-value	0,776	0,117	

Equal lower-case letters in the same column and upper-case letters in the same row indicate that there was no significant difference (p ≥ 0.05).

Contrary to what was observed in the OPG between adult and young animals, in the count of *Eimeria* sp. oocysts, it was found that animals up to 12 months old were the most parasitized. However, it was not possible to analyze this data statistically, as only one property had animals over 12 months old with an OOPG ≥ 2000 (table 6). As with the quantification of helminth eggs, it was possible to see a significant increase (*p* 0.0001) in relation to the established ranges of OOPG < 2000 and ≥ 2000 (table 6), in the two categories evaluated, also indicating high parasitism by *Eimeria* sp. in the region's animals.

Table 6. Count of *Eimeria sp.* oocysts per gram of feces (OoPG) on goat farms in the semi-arid region of Bahia.

	OOPG < 2000	OOPG ≥ 2000	p-value
Animals up to 12	475 ± 635 aA	21.960 ± 18290	0,0001

months	(n = 12)	*B (n = 5)
Animals ≥ 12 months	225 ± 217 a (n = 19)	2.100 ± 0 * (n = 1)
p-value	0,123	

Equal lower-case letters in the same column and upper-case letters in the same row indicate that there was no significant difference (p ≥ 0.05).

(*) Insufficient data to calculate statistically.

By analyzing the data obtained from the questionnaires, it was possible to draw up a profile of the farms, management techniques and producers' perceptions of the importance and methods of controlling gastrointestinal helminthiases and eimeria on the 20 farms studied (table 7).

Table 7. Quantitative characterization of dairy goat farms in the semi-arid region of Bahia.

Information from the owners	Responses in frequency order						
	1st place	%	2nd place	%	3rd place	%	N
Breeding System	Semi-intensive	80	Intensive	15	Extensive	5	20
Number of animals per property	26-50	55	0-25	40	More than 50	5	20
Water fountain	Supply company	50	Tank	45	Dam	5	20
Cleaning the drinking fountain	1 time a week	65	It doesn't	25	2 times a week	10	20
Product exchange	Base	70	Trademark	30	-	-	20
Knowledge about Eimeriosis	Yes	65	No	35	-	-	20
Drugs they used to Eimeriosis	Anti-helminthic	65	Coccidiostatic	35	-	-	20
Most commonly observed clinical signs	Diarrhea	50	Pallid mucous membranes	35	Oedemas	15	20

The main farming system in the region was semi-intensive (80%), followed by intensive

(15%) and the least common, extensive. Another profile found in the study was the number of goats per property, with the predominant range being 26 to 50 (55%), followed by properties with up to 25 animals (40%) and only 5% with more than 50 goats.

The main source of the water supplied to the animals on the farms was the local water company (50%), followed by tank water (45%) and, to a lesser extent, dam water (5%). Another factor, still in relation to the water supplied to the animals, was the frequency of cleaning the drinking troughs. It was found that the majority of owners cleaned them once a week (65%), but 25% said they didn't clean them often and 10% cleaned them twice a week.

When checking how anthelmintics were rotated on farms, it was found that 70% of producers changed the active ingredient, while 30% changed only the commercial brand. As a result of the correct need to rotate anthelmintics, this factor was associated with the most parasitized animals, i.e. those over 12 months of age (Table 8); however, there was no statistical difference between the factors analyzed.

Table 8. Influence of the rotation of drugs used to control gastrointestinal helminths on the egg count per gram of feces in animals over 12 months old.

	OPG < 800	OPG ≥ 800	Total	p-value (*)
Brand	3 (15%)	3 (15%)	6 (30%)	
Principle active	8 (40%)	6 (30%)	14 (70%)	1,000
Total	11 (69%)	9 (31%)	20 (100%)	

(*) No significant difference when p-value ≥ 0.05.

With regard to knowledge of eimeriosis, 65% of producers said they knew about it, but 35% did not. This factor was also analyzed statistically, but showed no significant difference (Table 9).

Table 9. Influence of the owners' knowledge of *Eimeria* on the count of *Eimeria* oocysts per gram of feces in animals under 12 months of age on goat farms in the semi-arid region of Bahia.

	OoPG < 2000	OoPG > 2000	Total	p-value
I knew Eimeriosis	8 (50%)	2 (13%)	10 (63%)	
I didn't know Eimeriosis	3 (19%)	3 (19%)	6 (37%)	0,299
Total	11 (69%)	5 (31%)	16 (100%)	

(*) No significant difference when p-value ≥ 0.05.

In order to assess how the treatment of eimeriosis was carried out on these properties, the type of medication used was questioned, and it was found that 65% of the producers treated their animals using anthelmintics and only 35% used coccidiostats. In the statistical analysis of this factor, no significant difference was found, but numerically it was possible to see that on most of the properties with the highest OoPGs, eimirosis was treated using anthelmintics (table 10).

Table 10. Influence of the medication used to control *Eimeria* on the count of *Eimeria* oocysts per gram of feces in animals under 12 months of age on dairy goat farms in the semi-arid region of Bahia.

	OoPG < 2000	OoPG > 2000	Total	p-value
Coccidiostàtico	4 (50%)	1 (13%)	5 (31%)	
Anti-helmitic	7 (44%)	4 (25%)	6 (69%)	1,000
Total	11 (69%)	5 (31%)	16 (100%)	

(*) No significant difference when p-value ≥ 0.05.

The most common clinical signs observed in the herds evaluated were diarrhea (50%), followed by pale mucous membranes (35%) and edema (15%), as mentioned above (Table 3). When analyzing the relationship between the most frequently observed clinical signs and the quantification of helminth eggs and *Eimeria* sp. oocysts in the animals, no significant differences were observed as the OPG and/or OoPG count increased (tables 11 and 12).

Table 11. Relationship between the frequency of clinical signs in animals over and under 12 months of age and the count of gastrointestinal helminth eggs per gram of feces in goat farms in the semi-arid region of Bahia.

	OPG of animals ≥ 12 months						p-value
	≥ 800		< 800		Grand total		
Pallid mucous membranes	n	%	n	%	n	%	
NO	6	66,67%	3	33,33 %	9	100%	**0,0813**
YES	2	18,18%	9	81,82 %	11	100%	
Diarrhea							
NO	3	50,00%	3	50,00 %	6	100%	**0,9207**
YES	5	35,71%	9	64,29 %	14	100%	

	OPG of animals under 12 months						p-value
	≥ 800		< 800		Grand total		
Pallid mucous	n	%	n	%	n	%	

membranes							
NO	3	33,33%	4	44,44 %	9	100%	**0,9731**
YES	4	36,36%	5	45,45 %	11	100%	
Diarrhea	2	33,33%	3				**0,9503**
NO				50,00 %	6	100%	
YES	5	35,71%	6	42,86 %	14	100%	

() There is no significant difference when the p-value is ≥ 0.05.

Table 12. Relationship between the frequency of clinical signs in animals over and under 12 months of age and the count of *Eimeria* sp. oocysts per gram of feces on dairy goat farms in the semi-arid region of Bahia.

	OoPG of animals ≥ 12 months						p-value
	≥ 2000		< 2000		Grand total		
Mucosa							
Pâlidas	n	%	n	%	n	%	
NO	1	11,11%	8	88,89%	9	100,00%	**0,9179**
YES	0	0,00%	11	100,00%	11	100,00%	
Diarrhea							
NO	1	16,67%	5	83,33%	6	100,00%	**0,6543**
YES	0	0,00%	14	100,00%	14	100,00%	

	OoPG of animals under 12 months old						p-value
	≥ 2000		< 2000		Grand total		
Mucosa							
Pâlidas	n	%	n	%	n	%	
NO	4	44,44%	3	33,33%	7	100,00%	**0,1414**
YES	1	9,09%	8	72,73%	9	100,00%	
Diarrhea							
NO	2	33,33%	3	50,00%	5	100,00%	**0,8502**
YES	3	21,43%	8	57,14%	11	100,00%	

7 - DISCUSSION

Parasitic gastroenteritis caused by helminths and eimeriosis are common in goats and can be considered the main health problems in goat farming (COSTA et al., 2009). As the northeast is the largest goat farming region in Brazil, these diseases have been widely studied (RIET-CORREA et al., 2013). In this study, the quantitative analysis of OPG and OoPG showed high counts of helminth eggs from the *Trichostrongyloidea* superfamily *and Eimeria* oocysts in all the properties analyzed. Corroborating these results, Ahid et al. (2008) also found a high rate of parasitism in small ruminants in the state of Rio Grande do Norte, through an analysis of 501 samples, where 71.2% were from goats and 25.7% from sheep, with 49.5% of the goats found to have gastrointestinal helminths and 41.3% being parasitized by *Eimeria.* With regard to age group, it was found that there was no significant difference between animals over 12 months old and young animals in the count of helminth eggs per gram of feces, however, the highest OPG values were observed in animals over 12 months old. According to Hoste et al (2010), infection levels in goats are similar in young and adult animals, but breeding females are more susceptible and have the highest parasite loads, especially primiparous females and also lactating females at the peak of lactation (HOSTE et al., 2002).

The quantification of *Eimeria* oocysts showed that young animals had a higher OoPG than adult animals, corroborating previous studies (FREITAS et al., 2005; BARBOSA et al., 2003; YOSOF ; ISA, 2016;). This greater susceptibility to *Eimeria* infection in young animals is due to the lack of prior immunity and also to the rapid proliferation of the protozoon (COSTA et al., 2009). However, it is worth noting that adult animals, even if they are immunologically competent, can be infected and continue to release oocysts in their feces, contaminating the environment and, above all, younger animals (AHID et al., 2008; KAHAN; GREINER, 2013).

The results obtained from the analysis of the questionnaires applied made it possible to understand the profile of the properties and the perception of dairy goat producers in the semi-arid region of Bahia regarding the methods of controlling worms and eimeria. In general, these are small farms, whose predominant farming method is semi-intensive, with between 26 and 50 animals in most flocks. This type of production is considered common in the Northeast of Brazil, providing a guarantee of family subsistence (AHID et al., 2008). However, this type of farming favors the maintenance of both worms and eimeria, since the animals spend some time together, due to the need for supplementation, thus facilitating the transmission of parasitic agents.

Anthelmintic control and the rotation of these drugs were carried out empirically on 100% of the farms, with 35% of the producers changing their anthelmintics only for the commercial brand. When analyzing the effect of how the choice of anthelmintic was made on the OPG value, no significant difference was found between the variables. However, the change of anthelmintic should be based on the active ingredient, since frequent and continued use of the same pharmacological base accelerates the selection process of resistant helminths (WALLER, 1994).

With regard to AR, it was possible to observe that 15% of the properties (3/20) had OPG results above the acceptable level in the period between 15 and 20 days after deworming with closantel and levamisole, which suggests that there is resistance to the anthelmintics used or high contamination of pastures with helminth larvae and/or hypobiosis (ARO et al., 2006).

Another relevant characteristic observed was that 35% of the producers in the study region did not know about eimeria, so they did not use coccidiostats and the animals were always treated with anthelmintics. In the statistical analysis to verify the association between these factors and the count of *Eimeria* oocysts, there was no significant difference, but there were more animals with OoPG above 2000 on properties where the owners did not know about eimeria and did not treat them correctly. According to Lima (2004), treatment should be carried out using specific drugs, the effectiveness of which depends on how early they are applied, as most of the drugs available for eimeria act on the early forms of coccidian multiplication. The most recommended drugs for the treatment of coccidiosis in ruminants are sulphas, amprolium, decoquinate, ionophoric antibiotics (monensin, salinomycin, lasalocid) and toltrazuril, as they are the active ingredients that show the best results (LIMA, 2004).

The most common clinical signs observed in the animals on the farms studied were diarrhea, pale mucous membranes and edema, but without exacerbated clinical manifestations. In addition, no significant difference was observed in the association of the parasite load of either gastrointestinal helminths or *Eimeria* with an increase in the frequency of clinical signs. According to Riet-Correa et al (2013), the presence of gastrointestinal parasites is constant, but with a high parasite load they can cause clinical disease. In general, worms and eimeria in goats are quite common in the northeast, where most animals are asymptomatic, so preventative measures should be adopted to minimize the spread of helminth eggs and coccidian oocysts. However, during field visits, some young animals showed clinical signs of diarrhea, weakness and anorexia, which could be associated with eimeria. This was also verified by Gazyagci et al. (2015) in a 1-month-old Saanen goat that died with similar symptoms and an oopg count of 9,900, with a predominance of the *E. arloingi* species. However, the absence of diarrhea in young goats does not rule out eimeria, given the results observed by these authors during their work.

The survival of larvae on pasture is subject to climatic factors, pasture management, among others. In the present study, it was possible to observe that the supply of diets rich in concentrate altered the consistency and characteristics of the feces, which were not in the form of sibalas but rather a fecal mass similar to that of cattle, which possibly, according to Almeida et al. (2005), would enable greater survival and migration of the larvae.

8 - CONCLUSION

Through this study, it can be concluded that gastrointestinal worms and eimeria are present in more than 80% of the leiteiros goat farms studied in the sisaleira region of Bahia and that the profile of the farms studied is consistent with the regional reality, where the majority are family subsistence farms with a small number of animals. The majority of producers still have little knowledge of gastrointestinal parasites, especially eimeria, and as a result, the forms of control used for these diseases in the region are not sufficient.

Therefore, other forms of management need to be implemented, given that even with the unfavorable climate for the cycles of these parasites, they still perpetuate themselves and cause serious problems in herds, demonstrating that verminosis and eimeriosis are undoubtedly the biggest problems faced by these producers. In view of this, further work to disseminate the biology, epidemiology, management and control of these parasitic agents is necessary and would be very useful to owners in the semi-arid region of Bahia in combating these very important parasites.

9 - FINAL CONSIDERATIONS

This study shows that verminosis and eimeriosis are diseases of great importance in goat farming in the northeast of Brazil.

It was possible to see that eimeriosis is the main disease affecting young goats up to two months of age, and that many producers are unaware of this disease, which is evident when eimeriosis is treated with dewormers, which have no effect on coccids.

With regard to survival, dissemination and parasite resistance, we can infer that, despite the semi-arid climate and high levels of sunshine, the larvae manage to survive, either in the feces or small plants around the reservoirs from where they are possibly ingested along with the forage.

The use of anthelmintics without criteria may be leading to the emergence of parasite populations resistant to various chemical compounds.

However, it is clear that the region's producers need assistance, especially in terms of information.

10 - BIBLIOGRAPHICAL REFERENCES

ABO-SHEHADA, M.; ABO-FARIEHA, H.A. Prevalence of *Eimeria* species among goats in northern Jordan. Small Ruminats Research, v.49, p.109-113, 2003.

ACOSTA, J.F. J et al. Improving resilience against natural gastrointestinal nematode infections in browsing kids during the dry season in tropical Mexico. Veterinary Parasitology, v. 135, p. 163-173, 2006.

AFZAN, M.Y., ISA, M.L. Prevalence of gastrointestinal nematodiasis and coccidiosis in goats from three selected farms in Terengganu, Malaysia. Asian Pacific Journal of Tropical Biomedicine, V. 6, P. 735-739, 2016.

AHID, S. M. M. et al. Species of the genus *eimeria* schneider, 1875 (*apicomplexa: eimeriidae*) in small ruminants in the western mesoregion of the state of Rio Grande do Norte, Brazil. Ciência Animal Brasileira, v. 10, n. 3, p. 984-989, jul./set. 2009.

AHID, S. M. M. et al. Gastrointestinal parasites in goats and sheep in the western region of Rio Grande do Norte, Brazil. Ciência Animal Brasileira , v. 9, n. 1, p. 212218, 2008.

ALMEIDA, L. R.; CASTRO, A. A.; SILVA, A. H. F. Development, survival and distribution of gastrointestinal nematodes of ruminants in the dry season of the Baixada Fluminense, RJ. Revista Brasileira de Parasitologia Veterinària,14, 3, 89-94 (2005).

ALTREUTHER, G. et al. Efficacy of emodepside plus toltrazuril suspension (Procox® oral suspension for dogs) against prepatent and patent infection with *Isospora canis and Isospora ohioensis* complex in dogs. Parasitology Research, v.109, p.9-20, 2011.

AMARANTE, A. F. T. Controle da Verminose Ovina, Revista CFMV Suplemento Técnico. Sâo Paulo, year 11, n, January to April, 2005.

ANDRADE JÛNIOR, A.L.F.; SILVA, P.C.; AGUIAR, E.M.; SANTOS, F.G.A. Use of coccidiostat in mineral salt DNA study on ovine eimeriosis. Revista Brasileira de Parasitologia Veterinària, v.21, n.1, p.16-21,2012.

AROSEMENA N.A.E., BEVILAQUA C.M.L., MELO A.C.F.L., GIRAO M.D. Seasonal variations of gastrointestinal nematodes in sheep and goats from semiarid areas in Brazil. Revue Medicine Veterinaire. 150: 873-87. 1999.

BARBOSA, P. B. B. M.; VIEIRA, L.S.; LEITE, A. I.; BRAGA, A. P. Species of the genus Eimeria Schneider, 1875 (Apicomplexa: Eimeriidae) parasitic on goats in the municipality of Mossoró, Rio Grande do Norte. Ciência Animal, v. 138, n. 2, p. 6572, 2003.

BENVENUTI, C.L. et al. Phenotypic characterization of mixed-breed goats infected with gastrointestinal nematodes. In: ZOOTEC, 2009, Aguas de Lindóia. Proceedings... Aguas de Lindóia - SP: ZOOTEC.2009.

BERGAMASCO, P.L.F. Universidade Estadual de Sao Paulo, Faculdade Ciências Agràrias e Veterinàrias, Jaboticabal. *Biològico*, Sao Paulo, v.77, Suplemento 2, p.1-235, 2015.

BIRGEL, D. B. et al. Evaluation of the erythrocyte picture and the repercussion of the anemic state on the leukogram of goats with gastrointestinal worms. Pesquisa Veterinària Brasileira 34(3):199-204,2014.

BORGES C.C.L. *In vitro* activity of anthelmintics on infective larvae of gastrointestinal nematodes of goats, using the quantitative coproculture technique (Ueno, 1995). Parasitologia Latinoamericana 58:142-147, 2003. FLAP.

BORGES S.L. et al. Anthelmintic resistance in goat herds in the Caatinga and Atlantic Forest biomes. Pesquisa Veterinària Brasileira, v. 35, p. 643-648, 2015.

BONFIM, T. C. B.; LOPES, C. W. G. Levantamento de parasitos gastrintestinais em caprinos da Regiao Serrana do Estado do Rio de Janeiro. Revista Brasileira de Parasitologia Veterinària, v. 3, n. 2, p. 119-124, 1994.

BOWMAN, D.D. In: Georgi's Parasitology for Veterinarians. (9th ed). Elsevier. 2010.

BRAGHIERI, A. et al. Effect of grazing and homeopathy on milk production and immunity of Merino derived ewes. Small Ruminant Research, v.69, p.95-102, 2007.

BRITO, D.R.B. et al. Gastrointestinal parasites in goats and sheep from the Alto Mearim and Grajaù micro-region, in the state of Maranhao, Brazil. Ciência Animal Brasileira, v. 10, n. 3, p. 967-974, 2009.

CHAGAS, A. C. S.; DOMINGUES, L. F.; GAiNZA, Y. A. Cartilha de vermifugaçao de ovinos e caprino./Dados eletrônicos- Sao carlos, SP: Embrapa Pecuària Sudeste, 2013.

CEZAR A.S., CATTO J.B. & BIANCHIN I. Alternative control of ruminant gastrointestinal nematodes: current situation and perspectives. Ciência Rural 38(7):2083- 2091, 2008.

COSTA, C. A. F.; VIEIRA, L. S. Control of gastrointestinal nematodes in goats and sheep in the state of Cearà. Sobral: EMBRAPA-CNPC. 6 p,1984 (EMBRAPA-CNPC. Comunicado Tècnico, 13).

COSTA JÙNIOR, G, S. et al. Effect of strategic deworming with an active ingredient based on ivermectin on the incidence of gastrointestinal parasites in the UFPI goat herd. Ciência Animal Brasileira, v. 6, n. 4, p. 279-286, 2005.

COSTA V.M.M., SIMOES S.V.D. & RIET-CORREA F. Control of gastrointestinal parasitosis in sheep and goats in the semi-arid region of northeastern Brazil. Pesquisa Veterinària Brasileira 31 (1):65-71,2011.

COSTA, V. M. M.; SIMOES, S. V. D.; RIET-CORREA, F. Parasitic diseases in ruminants in the Brazilian semi-arid region. Pesquisa Veterinària Brasileira, v. 29, n. 7, p. 563-568. 2009.

DAUGSCHIES, A.; NAJDROWSKI, M. Eimeriosis in cattle: Current understanding. Journal of Veterinary Medicine B, v.52, p.417-427, 2005.

DEL CACHO, E. et al. Effect of the quinolone coccidiostat decoquinate on the rearrangement of chromosomes of *Eimeria tenella*. International Journal for Parasitology, v.36, p.1515-1520, 2006.

DEMELER, J.; KUTTLER, U.; SAMSON-HIMMELSTJERNA, von G. Adaptation and evaluation of three different in vitro tests for the detection of resistance to anthelmintics in gastro intestinal nematodes of cattle. Veterinary Parasitology. v. 170, p. 61-70, 2010.

DIEHL, M.S.; ATINDEHOU, K.K.; TÉRÉ, H.; BETSCHART, B. Prospect for anthelminthic plants in the Ivory Coast using ethnobotanical criteria. Journal of Ethnopharmacology, v. 95, p. 277-284, 2004.

FOREYT, W.J. Coccidiosis and cryptosporidiosis in sheep and goats. Veterinary Clinics North Food Animal Practics, v.6, p.655-669, 1990.

FOX, M. T. Pathophysiology of infection with gastrointestinal nematodes in domestic ruminants: recent developments. Veterinary Parasitology, v. 72, n. 3-4, p. 285-308,1997.

FREITAS, F. L. C. et al. Species of the genus *Eimeria Schneider*, 1875 (Apicomplexa: Eimeriidae) in dairy goats kept in an intensive system in the region of Sâo José do Rio Preto, state of Sâo Paulo, Brazil. Revista Brasileira de Parasitologia Veterinària, v. 14, n. 1, p. 7-10, 2005.

GAZYAG, A. N. et al. Coccidiosis Due to *Eimeria arloingi* Infection in a Saanen Goat Kid. Research Journal for Veterinary Practitioners. V. 3 P. 29, 2015.

GALLIDIS, E.; ANGELOPOULOU, K; PAPADOPOULOS, E. First identification of benzimidazole resistant Haemonchus contortus in sheep in Greece. Small Ruminant Research,v. 106, p. 27-29, 2012.

GASBARRE, L.C.; LEIGH, E.A.; SONSTEGARD, T. Role of the bovine immune system and genome in resitance to gastrointetinal nematodes. Veterinary Parasitology, v. 98, p. 51-64, 2001.

GEORGE, S. D. et al. The comparative efficacy of abamectin, monepantel and an abamectin/derquantel combination against fourth-stage larvae of a macrocyclic lactone-resistant *Teladorsagia spp.* Isolate infecting sheep. Veterinary Parasitology, v. 188, n. 1-2, p. 190-193, 2012. doi:10.1016/j.vetpar.2012.03.001.

GITHIGIA, S.M.; WALLER, P.J.; HANSEN, J.W. Impact of gastrointestinal helminths on production in goats in Kenya. Small Ruminants Research, v.42, p.2129, 2001.

GONÇALVES, I. G.; ECHEVARRIA, F. A. M. Copper in the control of gastrointestinal worms in sheep. Ciência Rural, v. 34, n. 1, jan-feb, 2004

GORDON, H.M.; WHITLOCK, H.V. A new technique for counting nematode eggs in sheep faeces. Journal of the Commonwealth Scientific and Industrial Research Organization, v. 12, p. 50-52, 1939.

HART S. Effective and sustainable control of nematode parasites in small ruminants: The need to adopt alternatives to chemotherapy with emphasis on biologic control. 5th International Symposium on Goats and Sheep, Joao Pessoa, PB. (CD-ROM), 2011.

HOSTE H., LE FRILEUX Y. & POMMARET A. Comparison of selective and systematic treatments to control nematode infection of the digestive tract in dairy goats. Veterinary Parasitology. 106:345-355,2002b.

HOSTE H. et al. Goat- nematode interactions: think differently. Trends Parasitology. 26 (8):376-381, 2010.

HOSTE H. et al. Interactions between nutrition and gastrointestinal infections with parasitic nematodes in goats. Small Ruminants Research. 60:1415, 2005.

HOSTE, H. Adaptive physiological processes in the host during gastrointestinal parasitism. International Journal of Parasitology, v. 31, n. 3, p. 231-244, 2001. doi:10.1016/S0020-7519(00)00167-3.

HOSTE, H.; TORRES-ACOSTA, J. F. J.; AGUILAR CABALLERO, A. J. Nutrition-parasite interactions in goats: is immunoregulation involved in the control of gastrointestinal nematodes. Parasite immunology, v. 30, n.2, p. 79-88, 2008.

BRAZILIAN JOURNAL OF GEOGRAPHY AND STATISTICS. Rio de JaneiroJBGE, 2012. Municipal livestock production. Available at: < ftp://ftp.ibge.gov.br/Producao_Pecuaria/Producao_da_Pecuaria_Municipal/2013/ppm 2013.pdf >. Accessed on: November 10, 2016.

JÙNIOR, C. S. G. et al. Effect of strategic deworming with an active ingredient based on ivermectin on the incidence of gastrointestinal parasites in the UFPi goat herd. Ciência Animal Brasileira, v. 6, n. 4, p. 279-286, 2005.

KAPLAN, R.M. et al. Validation of the FAMACHA© eye color chart for detecting clinical anaemia in sheep and goats on farms in southern United States. Veterinary Parasitology, v.123, n.1, p.105-120, 2004.

KAHAN, T. B.; GREINER, E. C. Coccidiosis of Goats in Florida, USA. Open Journal of Veterinary Medicine, 2013, v. 3, p. 209-212, 2013.

KRZYZANIAK, E. L. Parasitology Workbook: Parasitological Examination. Marilia: University of Marilia, 2003. 12 f. Handout.

LIMA, J.D. Coccidiosis of domestic ruminants. Revista Brasileira de Parasitologia Veterinària, v.13, suplemento 1, p.9-13, 2004.

MACIEL, F. C.; NOGUEIRA, F. R. C.; AHID, S. M. M. Health management of goats and sheep. In: CONFESSOR JR., A. A. Criaçâo familiar de caprinos e ovinos no Rio Grande do Norte: Orientações para visualizaçâo do Negócio Rural. Natal: SINTEC, EMATER, EMBRAPA; EMPARN, p. 391-426, 2006.

MINAYO, M. C. S. O desafio do conhecimento: Pesquisa qualitativa em saù. 2. ed. Sâo Paulo - Rio de Janeiro: HUCITEC - ABRASCO, 1993. 289 p.

MOLENTO, M. B. Parasite control in the age of drug resistance and changing agricultural practices. Veterinary Parasitology. 163, 229-234, 2009.

MOLENTO M.B., TASCA C., FERREIRA M., BONONI R. & STECCA E. Famacha method as an individual clinical parameter of Haemonchus contortus infection in small ruminants. Ciencia Rural 34: 1139-1145, 2004.

POMPONET, A.S. From Consumption to the Market: Current Challenges for Goat Farming in the Semi-Arid Northeast of Bahia. Desenbahia Magazine, n°10. 2009.

PIENAR, J. G.; BASSON, P. A.; du PLEISSIS, J. L, et al: Experimental studies with Strongyloides papilosus in goats, Onderstepoort Journal Veterinary Research 66: 191, 1999.

PINHEIRO, D. N. S. Seroepidemiological Survey of Caprine Encephalitis Arthritis in the Sisaleira Region and Evaluation of Risk Factors. Dissertation (master's degree) Federal University of Recôncavo da Bahia, Center for Agricultural, Environmental and Biological Sciences. 2015.

PUGH, D.G. In: Clinica de caprinos e ovinos. Sâo Paulo: Roca 2004. p. 1-19.

RADOSTITS, O. M. et al. In: Clinica Veterinària: Um tratado de doenças dos bovinos, ovinos, suinos, caprinos e equinos. 9ª ed. Guanabara Koogan. Rio de Janeiro, RJ. p.778-791. 2002.

REIS I.F. Control of gastrointestinal nematodes in small ruminants: strategic method *versus* Famacha©. Master's dissertation in Veterinary Sciences, State University of Ceará, Fortaleza. 79p.2004.

RINALDI L. & CRINGOLI G. Parasitological and pathophysiological methods for selective application of anthelmintic treatments in goats. Small Ruminants Research. 103:18-22 Journal of Agriculture Research. 1:99-102, 2012

ROBERTS F.H.S.; O'SULLIVAN J.P. Methods for egg counts and larval cultures for strongyles infesting the gastro-intestinal tract of cattle. Australian Journal of Agricultural Research, v.1, p. 99-102, 1950.

SIDDIKI, A.Z.; KARIM, M.J.; CHAWDHURY, E.H. Sulfonamide resistance in chicken coccidiosis: a clinico-pathological study. Bangladesh Journal of Microbiology, v.25, n.1, p.60-64, 2008.

SILVA, R.M.; FACURY-FILHO, E.J.; SOUZA, M.F.; RIBEIRO, M.F.B.; Natural infection by *Eimeria spp.* in a cohort of lambs raised extensively in Northeast Brazil. Pesquisa Veterinària Brasileira. 20: 134-139, 2011.

SIMPLICIO, A. A. Goat and sheep farming: an alternative for generating employment and income. Available at: < http://www.cnpc.embrapa.br/artigo-6.htm >. Accessed on: November 3, 2016.

SOUZA, P. et al. Period for disinfection of pastures by sheep gastrointestinal nematode larvae, under natural conditions in the fields of Lages, SC. Revista Brasileira de Parasitologia Veterinària, Jaboticabal, v.9, p.159-164, 2000

SPRENGER, L. K. et al. Efficacy of levamisole phosphate on gastrointestinal nematodes of goats and sheep. Archives of Veterinary Science ISSN 1517- 784Xv.18, n.1, p.29-39, 2013

TERRILL, T. H. et al. Experiences with integrated concepts for the control of Haemonchus contortus in sheep and goats in the United States. Veterinary Parasitology, v.186, p.28- 37. 2012.

TIRABASSI, A. H. et al. Integrated parasite management as a sustainable alternative in small ruminant production Revista Acadêmica; Ciência Agrària Ambiental, Curitiba, v. 11, n. 3, p. 322-338, 2013.

TORRES-ACOSTA J.F.J. et al. Nutritional manipulation of sheep and goats for the control of gastrointestinal nematodes under hot humid and subhumid tropical conditions Small Ruminants Research. 103:28- 40.2012.

UENO, H.; GONÇALVES, P. C. In: Manual for the diagnosis of ruminant helminthiases. 4. ed. Tokyo: Japan International cooperation agency, 1998. 143p.

URQUHART, G. M. et al. In: Parasitologia veterinària. Rio de Janeiro: Guanabara Koogan, 1990. 306 p.

VIEIRA, L. da S.; CAVALCANTE, A. C. R.; XIMENES, L. J. F. Epidemiology and control of the main goat parasites in the semi-arid regions of Northeast Brazil. Sobral: Embrapa-CNPC, 1997. 50 p.

VIEIRA, L. S. Importance of gastrointestinal endoparasitosis in goat and sheep farming. In: SEMINARIO NORTE RIOGRANDENSE DE CAPRINOCULTURA E OVINOCULTURA, 1., 2005, Mossoró. Proceedings... Natal: UFERSA, SEBRAE-RN, CRMV-RN, 2005a CD-ROM

VIEIRA L.S. Alternative methods for controlling gastrointestinal nematodes in goats and sheep. Revista Ciência Tecnològica Agropecuâria. 2: p,28-31,2008.

WALLER, J.P. The development of anthelmintic resistance in ruminants. Acta tropica, v. 56, p. 233- 243, 1994.

YOUNG, G.; ALLEY, M.L.; FOSTER, D.M.; SMITH, G.W. Efficacy of amprolium for the treatment of pathogenic *Eimeria* species in Boer goat kids. Veterinary Parasitology, v.178, n.3-4, p.346-349, 2011.

11- ANNEXES

ANNEX I

Benzimidazole class anti-haemetics

Produto	Fabricante	Composição*	Indicação	Dose	Administração	Período de Carência (dias) Ovino Carne	Ovino Leite	Caprino Carne	Caprino Leite
Albemax 100	Vansil	Albendazol (10 g)	Ovi/Cap	0,4 mL/10 Kg PV	Oral	12	2	12	2
Albenda thor 10	Tortuga	Albendazol (10 g)	Ovi	0,5 mL/10 Kg PV	Oral	14	3	-	-
Albendazol Oral	Vittalfarma	Albendazol (10 g) + Cobalto (1,3 g)	Ovi/Cap	0,35 mL/10 Kg PV	Oral	14	Não tratar	ni	ni
Alabendazole 1,9% Labovet	Labovet	Albendazol (1,9 g)	Ovi/Cap	2 mL/10 KgPV	Oral	12	ni	12	ni
Alabendazole 10% Labovet	Labovet	Albendazol (10 g)	Ovi/Cap	0,4 mL/10 Kg PV	Oral	12	2	12	2
Aldazol 10 CO	Vallée	Albendazol (10 g) + Cobalto (1,3 g)	Ovi/Cap	0,5 mL/10 Kg PV	Oral	12	2	12	2
Bifetacol 10%	Microsules	Fenbendazol (10 g)	Ovi	0,5 mL/10 Kg PV	Oral	14	3	-	-
Bovalben	Vilavet	Albendazol (5 g)	Ovi/Cap	0,75 mL/10 Kg PV	Oral	14	2	14	2
Bovalben 10	Vilavet	Albendazol (10 g)	Ovi/Cap	0,4 mL/10 Kg PV	Oral	14	2	14	2
Calbendazole	Calbos	Albendazol (5 g)	Ovi /Cap	0,75 mL/10 Kg PV	Oral	14	3	14	3
Calbendazole 10%	Calbos	Albendazol (10 g)	Ovi	0,5 mL/10 Kg PV	Oral	10	ni	-	-
Endazol 10% Cobalto	Hipra	Albendazol (10 g) + Cobalto (1,3 g)	Ovi/Cap	0,35 mL/10 Kg PV	Oral	12	2	12	2
Farmazole ovinos 1,9%	Fagra	Albendazol (1,9 g)	Ovi/Cap	2 mL/10 KgPV	Oral	12	2	12	2
Fatoxen Oral	Alivet	Albendazol (10 g)	Ovi/Cap	0,5 mL/10 kg PV	Oral	14	3	14	3
Fencare 4% Premix	Virbac	Fenbendazol (4 g)	Ovi	1,25 g/10 kg PV	Na ração	15	ni	-	-
Ibazole 5%	Ibasa	Albendazol (5 g)	Ovi/Cap	0,8 mL/10 Kg PV	Oral	14	3	14	3
Ibazole 10%	Ibasa	Albendazol (10 g)	Ovi/Cap	0,4 mL/10 Kg PV	Oral	14	3	14	3
Magzole 5%	Leivas Leite	Albendazol (5 g)	Ovi	1 mL/10 Kg PV	Oral	12	2	-	-
Microparas 10% Oral	Microsules	Albendazol (10 g)	Ovi	0,5 mL/10 Kg PV	Oral	10	3	-	-
Oxfaden	Bio-Vet	Oxfendazol (2,26 g)	Ovi/Cap	1,1 mL/10 Kg PV	Oral	14	5	14	5
Panacur Suspensão	MSD	Fenbendazol (3 g)	Ovi/Cap	1,4 mL/10 kg PV	Oral	8	0	8	0
Pradozole 5%	Prado	Albendazol (5 g)	Ovi	0,75 mL/10 Kg PV	Oral	12	2	-	-
Provermin	Indubras	Fenbendazol (2 g)	Ovi/Cap	2,5 g/10 kg PV	Na ração ou água	14	3	14	3
Seguaymic Plus	Microsules	Triclabendazol (10 g) + Fenbendazol (10 g)	Ovi	1 mL/10 Kg PV	Oral	28	12	-	-
Valbazen 10% Cobalto	Pfizer	Albendazol (10 g) + Cobalto (1,3 g)	Ovi	0,5 mL/10 Kg PV	Oral	14	Não tratar	-	-
Waltec 10%	Dispeo do Brasil	Albendazol (10 g)	Ovi/Cap	0,4 mL/10 Kg PV	Oral	14	3	14	3

Source: Sheep and goat deworming booklet (EMBRAPA , 2013).

ANNEX II

Imidothiazole class anti-haemetics

Produto	Fabricante	Composição	Indicação	Dose	Administração	Período de Carência (dias) Ovino Carne	Ovino Leite	Caprino Carne	Caprino Leite
Adevermin	Fagra	Cloridato de tetramisol (10 g) + vit. A, D, E e anti-histamínico	Ovi/Cap	0,7 mL/10 kg PV	SC, IM	ni	ni	ni	ni
Bokill	Biofarm	Fosfato de levamisol (22,3 g)	Ovi/Cap	0,2 mL/10 kg PV	SC	ni	ni	ni	ni
Biopersol Forte MV	Biogénesis Bagó	Fosfato de levamisol (23,63 g)	Ovi	0,2 mL/10 kg PV	SC, IM, IP, IR	7	ni	-	-
Levamisol Calbos	Calbos	Cloridrato de levamisol (8 g)	Ovi/Cap	0,75 mL/10 kg PV	SC, IM	7	2	7	2
Levamisol Injetável	Noxon	Fosfato de levamisol (22,3 g)	Ovi	0,2 mL/10 kg PV	SC/IM	7	2	-	-
Levamil F-15	Fagra	Fosfato de levamisol (22,3 g)	Ovi	0,2 mL/10 kg PV	SC, IM	ni	ni	-	-
Protali VP	Vallée	Fosfato de levamisol (18,8 g)	Ovi/Cap	0,33 mL/10 kg PV	SC	7	2	7	2
Ripercol L Solução	Fort Dodge	Cloridato de levamisol (5 g)	Ovi	1 mL/10 kg PV	Oral	ni	ni	-	-
Vermicol	Vilavet	Cloridato de levamisol (8 g)	Ovi/Cap	0,5 mL/10 kg PV	SC	7	2	7	2

Source: Sheep and goat deworming booklet (EMBRAPA , 2013).

ANNEX III

Organophosphate class antihemetics

Produto	Fabricante	Composição	Indicação	Dose	Administração	Ovino		Caprino	
						Carne	Leite	Carne	Leite
Ciclosom	Leivas Leite	Triclorfon (50 g) + Sulfato de atropina	Ovi	0,66 mL/10 kg PV	SC, IM	ni	1	-	-
Ibafon	Ibasa	Triclorfon (50 g) + Sulfato de atropina	Ovi/Cap	0,5 mL e 0,66 mL /10 kg PV	SC	7	ni	7	ni
Neguvon	Bayer	Triclorfon (97 g)	Ovi/Cap	10 mL de sol. a 10%/10 kg PV	oral	7	1/2	7	1/2
Triclorfon 97%	Vitalfarma	Triclorfon (97 g)	Ovi/Cap	10 mL de sol. a 10%/10 kg PV	oral	7	1	7	1
Triclorsil	Vansil	Triclorfon (98 g)	Ovi/Cap	10 mL de sol. a 10%/10 kg PV	oral	7	1	7	1
Triveron	Allvet	Triclorfon (20 g)	Ovi/Cap	5 mL/10 kg PV	oral	7	2	7	2

Source: Sheep and goat deworming booklet (EMBRAPA , 2013).

ANNEX IV

Salicylanilide class antihemetics and phenolic substitutes

Produto	Fabricante	Composição	Indicação	Dose	Administração	Ovino		Caprino	
						Carne	Leite	Carne	Leite
Allpar	Hipra	Closantel (10 g) + Albendazol (3.8 g)	Ovi	1 mL/10 kg PV	Oral	30	30	-	-
Closalben	Vetbrands	Closantel (7.5 g) + Albendazol (3.8 g)	Ovi/Cap	1 mL/ 10 Kg PV	Oral	14	Não tratar	14	Não tratar
Diantel 10%	Hipra	Closantel (10 g)	Ovi/Cap	1 mL/10 kg PV	Oral	30	30	30	30
Disofen 20	Champion	Disofenol (20 g)	Ovi	0,5 mL/10 kg PV	SC	zero	2	-	-
Disofenol 20%	Ibasa	Disofenol (20 g)	Ovi/Cap	0,5 mL/10 kg PV	SC	zero	2	zero	2
Dovenix Supra	Merial	Nitroxinil (34 g)	Ovi/Cap	0,3 mL/10 kg PV	SC	30	Não Tratar	30	Não Tratar
Galgosantel oral 7.5	Biogénesis Bagó	Closantel (7,5 g)	Ovi	1 mL/10 kg PV	Oral	28	14	-	-
Microtel Bovinos, Ovinos e Equinos	Microsules	Closantel (10 g) + Albendazol (5 g)	Ovi	1 mL/10 kg P/	Oral	30	Não Tratar	-	-
Nitromic	Microsules	Nitroxinil (34 g)	Ovi	0,2 mL/10 kg PV	SC	60	Não Tratar	-	-
Nitroxynil Fina	Champion	Nitroxinil (34 g)	Ovi	0,6 mL/10 kg PV	SC	30	3	-	-
Pradoverme	Prado	Disofenol (10 g) + Cloridrato de tetramisol (8 g)	Ovi/Cap	0,66 mL/10 kg PV	SC/IM	14	3	14	3
Rumivac 30	Champion	Disofenol (30 g)	Ovi	0,25 mL/10 kg PV	SC	zero	2	-	-
Rumivac 1/10	Champion	Disofenol (8 g)	Ovi	1 mL/10 kg PV	Oral	ni	2	-	-
Rumivac 1/20	Champion	Disofenol (10 g)	Ovi	0,5 mL/10 kg PV	Oral	ni	2	-	-
Taitec Oral	Calbos	Closantel (10 g)	Ovi	0,5 mL/10 kg PV	Oral	15	15	-	-
Zuletel 10% injetável	Microsules	Closantel (10 g)	Ovi	0,5 mL/10 kg PV	SC	42	Não Tratar	-	-
Zuletel 10%	Microsules	Closantel (10 g)	Ovi	0,5 mL/10 kg PV	Oral	30	30	-	-

Source: Sheep and goat deworming booklet (EMBRAPA , 2013)

ANNEX V

Avermectin class anthelmintics

Produto	Fabricante	Composição	Indicação	Dose	Administração	Ovino		Caprino	
						Carne	Leite	Carne	Leite
Aba-Allvet LA	Eurofarma	Abamectina (1 g)	Ovi	0.2 mL/10 kg PV	SC	49	Não tratar	-	-
Absolut	Vallée	Ivermectina (1 g) + vitaminas, aminoácidos e minerais	Ovi/Cap	0.2 mL/10 kg PV	SC	28	Não tratar	28	Não tratar
Alteo	Tortuga	Ivermectina (1 g)	Ovi/Cap	0.2 mL/10 kg PV	SC	28	Não tratar	28	Não tratar
Avotan LA	MSO	Abamectina (1 g)	Ovi/Cap	0.2 mL/10 kg PV	SC, IM	42	Não tratar	42	Não tratar
Bullmec Clássico	Clarion	Ivermectina (1 g)	Ovi	0.2 mL/10 kg PV	SC	28	ni	-	-
Dectomax	Pfizer	Doramectina (1 g)	Ovi	0.2 mL/10 kg PV	SC, IM	35	Não tratar	-	-
Doractin injetável	Vitalfarma	Doramectina (1 g)	Ovi	0.2 mL/10 kg PV	SC, IM	ni	ni	-	-
Doramec	Eurofarma	Doramectina (1 g)	Ovi	0.2 mL/10 kg PV	SC, IM	35	ni	-	-
Exceller	Vallée	Doramectina (1 g)	Ovi	0.2 mL/10 kg PV	SC, IM	35	Não tratar	-	-
Ivergold	Prado	Ivermectina (1 g)	Ovi	0.2 mL/10 kg PV	SC	35	Não tratar	-	-
Ivermax	Dispec do Brasil	Ivermectina (1 g)	Ovi	0.2 mL/10 kg PV	SC	21	ni	-	-
Ivermectan	UCB Saúde nimal	Ivermectina (1 g)	Ovi/Cap	0.2 mL/10 kg PV	SC	21	Não tratar	21	Não tratar
Ivermectina OF	Ouro Fino	Ivermectina (1 g)	Ovi	0.2 mL/10 kg PV	SC	28	Não tratar	-	-
Ivermic 1%	Microsules	Ivermectina (1 g)	Ovi	0.2 mL/10 kg PV	SC	28	Não tratar	-	-
Ivermic + ad3e	Microsules	Ivermectina (1.1 g) + vitaminas	Ovi/Cap	0.2 mL/10 kg PV	SC	28	Não tratar	28	Não tratar
Ivermic Oral 0.2%	Microsules	Ivermectina (0.2 g)	Ovi/Cap	1 mL/10 kg PV	Oral	14	Não tratar	14	Não tratar
Ivergen	Biogénesis Bagó	Ivermectina (1 g)	Ovi	0.2 mL/10 kg PV	SC	ni	ni	-	-
Ivomec Injetável	Merial	Ivermectina (1 g)	Ovi	0.2 mL/10 kg PV	SC	28	Não tratar	-	-
Ivomec Sol. Oral	Merial	Ivermectina (0.08 g)	Ovi/Cap	2.5 mL/10 kg PV	Oral	11	Não tratar	21	Não tratar
Leivamec	Leivas Leite	Ivermectina (1 g)	Ovi	0.2 mL/10 kg PV	SC	28	Não tratar	-	-
Mogimec	Bimeda Mogivet	Ivermectina (1 g)	Ovi	0.2 mL/10 kg PV	SC	28	Não tratar	-	-
Ranger	Vallée	Ivermectina (1 g)	Ovi/Cap	0.2 mL/10 kg PV	SC	28	Não tratar	28	Não tratar
Ranger LA	Vallée	Ivermectina (1 g)	Ovi/Cap	0.2 mL/10 kg PV	SC, IM	42	Não tratar	42	Não tratar

Source: Sheep and goat deworming booklet (EMBRAPA , 2013).

ANNEXVI

Amino-acetonitrile Derivatives (AADs) antihemetics

Produto	Fabricante	Composição	Indicação	Dose	Administração	Período de Carência (dias)			
						Ovino		Caprino	
						Carne	Leite	Carne	Leite
Zolvix	Novartis	Monepantel (2.5 g)	Ovi	1 mL/10 kg PV	Oral	7	Não tratar	-	-

Source: Sheep and goat deworming booklet (EMBRAPA , 2013).

ANNEX VII- Antiprotozoals (Non-sulfamides and sulfamides)

Base Pharmacology	Trade name	Dose mg/kg	Via		Duration	Source:
Sulfadoxine w/ trimethoprim	w/	15	IV1 IM1 SC	12 24		Radostits et al., 2002
Sulfonamide trimethoprim	/	15-30	IV,IM	12 24		Radostits et al.1 2002
Sulfaquinoxaline	®trissufin	15-30 (25)	VO	24	3 -5 days	Radostits et al.1 2002
Sulfamethoxypyridazina		20	SC1IM1IV	24		Radostits et al.1 2002
Sulfadiazine		15-30	VO	24		Radostits et al.1 2002
Monesina		20 g/ton (1mg/cab/day)	VO	24		Bowman1 2010
Lasolacid		20-30 g/ton (15-70 mg/cab/day) 0.5	VO	24		Bowman1 2010
Decoquinate			VO	24	28 days	Bowman1 2010
Amprolio		55	VO	12	19 days	Bowman1 2010
Toltrazuril	®Baycox	20	VO	24	Single dose	Bula

Questionnaire applied to producers.

FEDERAL UNIVERSITY OF RECONCAVO DA BAHIA CENTER OF AGRICULTURAL, ENVIRONMENTAL AND BIOLOGICAL SCIENCES FINAL COURSE WORK
Name:
Municipality   tel:
Ownership:
He lives on the property: Total area:
Cultivated pasture:
Pasture rotation: Occupation time:
Mineralization: Supplementation:
Aprisco: Yes (   ) No ( ) Type: Rammed ( ) Cemented ( ) Ripped ( )
Total number of animals: Breeds:
Breeding system: Intensive (   )   semi-intensive (   )   extensive (   )
Separate lots by age: Yes ( )   No (   )
Cleaning drinking fountains and feeders:
Destination of feces:
Main herd health problems:
( ) Diarrhea in adults   (   ) Low weight gain
( ) Diarrhea in young people   (   )Anemia,   bocabranca
( ) Submandibular   edema   (   )Intolerance   exercise
( ) Youth mortality   (   ) Adult   mortality
( ) Lymphadenitis   (   )Verminosis
( ) Ecthyma contagiosum   (   )Eimeriosis
( )Mastitis   (   ) Ectoparasites (lice, ticks)
In the event of death, the clinical signs presented:
Do you know Eimeriosis: Yes (   ) No (   ) What Treatment:
Vaccines: Clostridiosis   () Rabies ( ) Lymphadenitis( ) others:
Worming the animals: Yes (   )   No (   )
How many times a year:
Last deworming :   Product:
Dosage: Package   insert(   )Other Owner() Seller (   ) Veterinarian( )
Worming rotation: Yes (   ) No () / Active ingredient (   )   Brand (   )
Do Opg/   OopgYes ( )   No (   ) Last time:

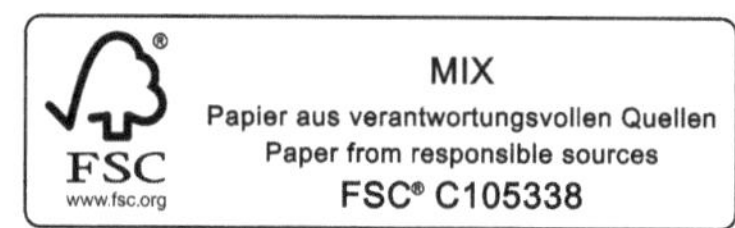

Printed by Books on Demand GmbH, Norderstedt / Germany